The Mad Cow Crisis
Health and the Public Good

Edited by

Scott C. Ratzan

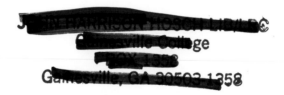
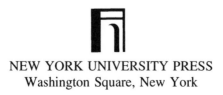

NEW YORK UNIVERSITY PRESS
Washington Square, New York

First published in the U.S.A. in 1998 by
NEW YORK UNIVERSITY PRESS
Washington Square
New York, N.Y. 10003

Library of Congress Cataloging-in-Publication Data
The mad cow crisis : health and the public good / edited by Scott C.
   Ratzan.
      p.   cm.
   ISBN 0-8147-7510-1 (hbk.). – ISBN 0-8147-7511-X (pbk.)
   1. Bovine spongiform encephalopathy—Social aspects.   2. Bovine
spongiform encephalopathy—Political aspects.   3. Mass media in
health education.   4. Creutzfeldt—Jacob disease—Social aspects.
5. Creutzfeldt–Jacob disease—Political aspects.   I. Ratzan, Scott
C.
RA644.P93M33   1998
362.1'9683–dc21   97-38913
                                                                              CIP

Printed in Great Britain

Preface

Humankind has reached a point at the end of the twentieth century at which "science" is expected to have explanations for everything. "Scientifically proven" theories are seen as progress by a public hungry for information on how to obtain good health and longevity. Each week a new study proclaims that something we eat or drink (beef, coffee, alcohol); something we do (over-work, use cellular phones); or things which we cannot control (for example our genetic make-up) are responsible for disease, premature ageing, or other calamities. The information disseminated from reports in the media instantly becomes "factual" as we, in turn, repeat what we have heard or read with the omnipotent "they say". We than make individual decisions on how to react based on what "they" suggest we do.

Over a century ago, James Fenimore Cooper first warned, " 'They say' is the monarch of this country, in a social sense. No one asks '*who* says it', so long as it is believed that '*they* say it'." Today, "they say" is of even greater importance than it was in James Fenimore Cooper's time. The world is more complicated, and "they" have the power to communicate instantaneously throughout the world and have a huge impact on our everyday lives.

The mad cow crisis is arguably one of the greatest human-made disasters in history. Initially, the British Government revealed that there might be links between a fatal disease termed bovine spongiform encephalopathy (BSE), or mad cow disease, and human deaths. While direct and immediate human deaths are not immediately evident, the $10 billion or more that it has cost rank it alongside other human-made disasters such as the *Exxon Valdez*, Chernobyl or Bhopal.

This book presents a multi-disciplinary approach to the crisis, with viewpoints from experts across a variety of fields, in an attempt to comprehend the ramifications of this unique case. This study covers the history of the crisis which nobody wished to claim as their own. The medical community called the disease a veterinary issue whilst the veterinarians claimed it a government/ public health issue. Both the UK and European governments, having no clear communication strategy, acknowledged it as a scientific dilemma. They both used science subjectively, blaming the media and each other for the escalation of the crisis. The media was keen to keep the story in the public's mind with political and medical reporters vying to present the lead story. The principal contribution of the academic and scientific community was in producing one after another study in support or against the hypothesis of the microscopic nature of the disease and the potential rationale for the 12 new cases of CJD (Creutzfeldt–Jakob disease) and the epidemiological ramifications. Conjecture and "what if" scenarios became ubiquitous.

Warnings were made of the inadequate preparation for such crises and clearly the mad cow crisis has evolved into a classic example of the demand for communications and leadership from those in the non-scientific community.

Whilst my expertise lies in the effective communication of health and risk issues, this book grew from my increasing interest in the disclosure from the Spongiform Encephalopathy Advisory Committee (SEAC) of a potential link between mad cow disease and human CJD deaths, released in March 1996. This development would obviously lead to a major international crisis. I quickly put my ideas and warnings in writing which culminated in an article in the *Boston Globe* in April 1996 entitled "Mad cow hysteria". Subsequent ideas were explored at a conference in Oxford and in articles in the *Journal of Health Communication*, the *Financial Times* and the *Wall Street Journal*.

The value of this book lies not only in a presentation of different views of the mad cow debate but also offers an understanding of how "they say that eating beef can kill you" becomes a "truism" in public minds. A chronology and media analysis chronicles the crisis in terms of the public's perception of science. There are also strategies for approaching events which involve health, risk and crisis that should be of particular value to readers involved in policy-making.

Finally, in recent years, interest in the subject of communicating health and risk has increased considerably. A recent World Health Organization (WHO) initiative is developing a strategy to deal with this issue as well as implementing training on national and international levels. I hope that this book will stimulate a more thorough examination of the subject of communicating health and risk so that we can manage future crises. Whilst presenting a number of viewpoints, this text should serve to make the reader question assumptions and balance sense with science. It will help the reader ask questions in the following vein: who are "they" and how worthy are they of our immediate respect? Why are "they" saying what they are and on what authority? It should also help the reader devise a plan to become the "they" in future for their respective public(s). Finally, it should help advance an ideal for a public literacy and responsible proactive policies so that "they say" will not threaten the societal progress of what we know.

Acknowledgments

Clearly, any edited volume requires a unique mix of contributions. I was fortunate in having an excellent set of contributors on both sides of the Atlantic who understood the objective of the book and could offer unique expertise. Each of the chapters has great value in adding to the comprehension of this complicated issue. In fact, many of the contributors look forward to examining the disparate views and different perspectives of their colleagues. Certain authors should be recognized for their help with the project beyond their single chapter, including Michael Chamberlain, Catherine Goethals and Michael Levy.

My background affords me a unique opportunity to serve on the faculty of Emerson College and Tufts University School of Medicine. As such, I have been lucky to discuss this project with various colleagues for whose support I am grateful: Cara Birritierri, Jim Hyde, Barry Levy, Jeanne Goldberg, Walt Littlefield, J. Gregory Payne, Morton Madoff, Mary Joyce, Norma Stearns, and Jim Tillotson.

Additionally, I often work with government agencies throughout the world on health, risk and communication issues, I am indebted to the insights and input certain experts in the field have shared with me: Barry Johnson, Maria Pavlova, Tim Tinker, Bernard Goldstein, Max Lum, and Chris Schonwalder in the US, Dick Mayon-White of the UK, as well as Carlos Dora and Franklin Apfel of the World Health Organization.

I am also happy to continue the relationship as editor-in-chief of the *Journal of Health Communication* published by Taylor & Francis. Their teams in the UK and US – Richard Steele, Alison Chapman, Bev Acreman – were instrumental in the Oxford conference and the initial phase of the project. The UCL Press editors Caroline Wintersgill, Fiona Kinghorn, and Mitch Fitton also contributed greatly to the quality of this project.

The editorial board of the *Journal of Health Communication* has shared its expertise not only with policy and editorial issues related to the journal, but also in its support of such multidisciplinary projects. I am indebted to particular board members – Tom Backer, Mary Jo Deering, Fred Kroger, Karen Hein, Everett Rogers, Vicki Freimuth, Bill Smith and Larry Wallack – for the support and time they have shared in advancing my career contribution.

Acknowledgments

In my principal position as director of the Emerson-Tufts Program in Health Communication – that has had over 100 students enrolled for a masters degree – I have benefited from student support and ideas. In particular, research fellow Veronica (Nicky) Demko has been instrumental in the success of this project. Her attention to detail and assimilation of not only the components of the book but also the compilation of the timeline is of great value. Other scholars in health communication – Holly Massett, Kari Kilroy, Angela Porter, Dan Dornbusch, Elizabeth Jack, Suzanne Meadows Hogan, Anne Restino, Carrie Stett and Amy Schmitz also deserve special mention for their input to this and other projects.

Also, the early development and support to continue this project could not have been accomplished without Shawn Donnelley, with her faxes and clips sent daily from around the world. Her additional support in the development of the Center for Ethics in Political and Health Communication at Emerson College helped advance the requisite ethical and objective focus of academic study.

I am neither a veterinarian, nor a beef farmer, nor a politician with a career at stake in the mad cow issue. But my interest in this case, and my professional development in medicine, government and communication, have grown from the ideals instilled in me by my parents, Jerry and Dawne Ratzan: to seek the truth, to distinguish between right and wrong, and to discriminate among values. My sister, Tami, and I have both benefited from their support and instruction. I hope that this book will do their teaching justice, in advancing the ideals of health for the next millennium.

Introduction

Scott C. Ratzan

> If one wanted an illustration of the manifold perils of imperfect policymaking, this case provides them all ... (*Guardian*, 30 May 1996)

The chronological development of the mad cow crisis presents a quintessential case in which scientists, politicians and representatives of the media responded to uncertainty and created the public meaning and understanding of a complicated issue.

In 1996, the BSE (bovine spongiform encephalopathy) issue erupted into a media melee, triggering public alarm and governmental wrangling that threatened the future of European integration and the health of the public. While hindsight revealed leadership to be lacking, the public yearned for accurate information related to their most precious resource – their health. The rhetorical ping-pong match of who would emerge with responsible leadership highlights the uncertainty surrounding the issue. The medical community labeled mad cow disease a veterinary issue. Veterinarians described it as a government/public health issue. The Government, in turn, with no clear communication strategy, termed it as a scientific dilemma and blamed the media for sensationalism. The media, keen to report in the competitive market struggle for a lead story, focused on questionable causal links and the politics of the situation rather than delving into the scientific grounds. The scientists, those who had objective "knowledge", were relegated to the laboratory while politicians and self-anointed "experts" in the media served as conduits to the public's understanding of this complicated scientific issue. All of this resulted in a crisis of confidence. The entire British beef industry faced devastating destruction. Trust in the quality of information waned.

The result of this lack of leadership: since the crisis began, hundreds of thousands of cattle have been slaughtered, farmers have lost their livelihood, the British Government is at odds both domestically and with Europe, the European Union is in a precarious position, engaged in new policies, and scientists continue to try to build upon actual "knowledge" in the effort to present evidence of *any* link to human death from ingestion of beef.

I began following this case in great depth immediately upon the announcement of the Spongiform Encephalopathy Advisory Committee (SEAC) report on 20 March 1996 and the subsequent coverage throughout the world. This initiated the drafting of an op-editorial for the *Boston Globe* highlighting the problems with the initial announcement of the BSE crisis and the probable ramifications of the government report which lacked any plan of response (I still stand by my initial response published in April). Although this issue had the potential to be addressed with appropriate crisis communication strategies, it was no surprise to me that it continued to spiral out of control. While in Brussels teaching a course in international negotiation and directing a health communication institute in summer, 1996, I had the opportunity to follow its escalation. I later presented the initial findings at the University of Oxford at a symposium entitled "High stakes in health communication: the mad cow issue". The idea for this book was initiated by the hearty discussions in Brussels and Oxford.

Earlier this century, Oxford's Regius Professor of Medicine, Sir William Osler reminded of the role of the physician: "The physicians' challenge is the curing of disease, educating the people in the laws of health and preventing the spread of plagues and pestilence" (Bean & Bean 1968: 63). As a physician and the son of a physician, throughout my entire life I have witnessed the changing role of the health care and the need for the optimal application of Osler's challenge. I have attempted to maximize my role as citizen and doctor to affect the public health through accurate communication to prevent disease and help create an environment for a healthier life. Whereas the effective communication of health is the focus of the masters program I direct and the *Journal of Health Communication* I edit, the mad cow issue had ramifications worthy of a special book for those interested in the progress of humankind.

As the twentieth century draws to a close with progress in science and humanities advancing at an ever-growing pace, health information still diffuses into the public mind amongst a variety of sources creating understanding and beliefs. In this fast-paced society the public often rushes to judgment on limited data and evidence formulating the omnipresent "they say" – a new, modern-day epistemology. "They say" is advanced with a new ethos through word of mouth, expression of images in the mass media, and through repetition.

While the case will continue to have an effect on politicians, policy-making and the public, it gives us the opportunity to examine the multidisciplinary understanding of an issue that escalated into what the European Commissioner for Agriculture, Franz Fischler, explained as "the biggest crisis the European Union had ever had". The beef crisis' economic cost to the European Union has exceeded $2.8 billion in 1996 alone.

This case serves as the focal point for a multidisciplinary approach in this book, *The mad cow crisis: health and the public good*. Several experts, principally from the United Kingdom and the United States, explain this crisis from unique vantage points with health and the public good as the underlying theme. This book does not attempt to present the scientific debate in detail, although it does elucidate how the imprecise nature of science can convolute a public thirst for accurate information.

Those in the fields of public health, communication, public relations, sciences, economics, government, mathematics, veterinary medicine, public administration, politics, psychology, infectious disease, negotiation, nutrition, medicine, public policy, and sociology, among other areas should find this book of interest. All those interested in how we reach an understanding of "health as we know it" should find this case fascinating, and can gain from the different perspectives offered by the authors.

The contents in this book are divided into four major sections: Scientific/historical perspectives, Politics as health, Understanding the crisis, and Lessons and possibilities. Following the authored sections is an extensive appendix including a timeline, governmental reports from throughout the world, and other materials.

The first section provides the foundation for the understanding of the crisis from a variety of perspectives addressing what *Nature* highlighted as a challenge: "And where mechanisms are poorly understood and epidemiological data sparse, as is the case in the various types of Creutzfeldt–Jakob Disease and the associated prion hypothesis, then it is inevitable that scientific judgement is uncomfortably imprecise" [*sic*] (2 January 1997, **385**: 1).

The Scientific/historical perspectives are approached with different disciplinary presentations. The understanding of science in the quest toward truth requires the artistic act to discriminate among values in quantification and objective description of "knowledge". Hence, this section includes articles from observers in the US including Lester Crawford (Executive Director of the Association of American Veterinary Colleges), neurological surgeons Michael Levy and Terri Harpold (Los Angeles Children's Hospital/University of Southern California School of Medicine) and Eve Brouwer (National Safety Council), as well as UK experts, microbiologist Steven Dealler (author of *Lethal legacy*), and Paul Anand (Wolfson College, University of Oxford) who termed the mad cow issue "the AIDS crisis the UK never had". These five chapters address the issue from multiple perspectives with models from mathematics, neurohistology, medicine, public health, anthropology, history, economics, and veterinary science.

The section Politics as health outlines the important relationship of how health issues escalate beyond the laboratory or within the confines of family decision making. Ian Wylie (Kings Fund, UK) highlights the early British dissemination of information and the politics behind the scenes. Dick Mayon-White (Oxfordshire Health Authority), who referred to himself as the "crisis doc" at the University of Oxford conference, describes the stages of the crisis, and the interface of government, science and the public. Professor of Food Policy, Tim Lang (Thames Valley University, Wolfson School of Health Sciences), one of the foremost professors who was selected by the British Government to draft a definitive memorandum on the crisis, shares this memorandum offering information on optimal policy formulation in a political world. Finally, Catherine Goethals (College of Europe) in consultation with Veronica Demko and myself, presents a European view of the negotiation and entangling interests in this case. Member of Parliament Simon Hughes (Liberal Democrat Health Spokesman) offers advice on how Britain should adapt the governmental structure to prepare and deal with a future mad ????? crisis and protect the public health. Much of the information in this section is gathered through interviews with various individuals and leaders who offered information on and off the record in an effort to help explain for the first time the rationale for decisions and reasoning behind the scenes. This section should be of interest not only to those who have followed the crisis, but also to all who would like to avert a crisis in the future and help predict the escalating flash points.

The section Understanding the crisis explores the process of how most of us gather information through the popular media sources. Science communication expert Joan Leach (Imperial College of London and Editor of *Social Epistemology*) suggests that much of what we know about the mad cow issue is a metaphor of meaning from the television coverage and popular culture representation of "mad cows". However, because much of the information we receive is generally derived from an agenda set by the print journalist, an extensive analysis of the press coverage in the United States is offered by research fellow Veronica Demko (Emerson–Tufts Program in Health Communication). Press coverage of over 400 articles in the most widely read newspaper in the world, the *Financial Times*, is offered by Dan Dornbusch (also of the Emerson–Tufts Program in Health Communication). J. Gregory Payne (director of the Center for Ethics in Political and Health Communication at Emerson College) places such coverage in a context of understanding the creation of a mediated reality.

The section Lessons and possibilities provides the reader with mechanisms to plan effectively for any crisis. Former journalist and new media expert, Michael Chamberlain (Informed Sources International Ltd) suggests the "tool box" of new media technologies available to help avert, avoid and manage a crisis. Dawn Hopkins (World Wildlife Fund) and Marcie Everett-Weber in Ottawa, Canada, present de-intensification of cattle farming and alternative policy approaches to avert disaster. Finally, I present four methodologies prevalent in strategic use of health communication – social marketing, public relations, negotiation, and advocacy – as integrated strategies for dissemination of health messages to target audiences.

The final section of the book, the Appendix, is meant as a resource to assist in the understanding of a complex issue with material from a variety of sources. The timeline provides a quick opportunity for case analysis, while the selection of government reports provides the official response to the crisis in government papers and proclamations along with other supplementary materials. The section should be of great value for the student, researcher, practitioner, and scholar.

It is the author's hope that the readers of this book will be able to understand the complexity of an issue that can have a great impact on everyone's lives. At the same time, the book should encourage the reader to question assumptions and to seek knowledge and understanding beyond the modern-day media experts, incremental subjective scientific suggestions, and political proclamations. It should also remind all of us of the need for a special kind of preparedness in an increasingly complex world so that we can work proactively and reactively with multidisciplinary approaches to help advance societal understanding and decisions on issues that affect the public good.

Scott C. Ratzan
March 1997

References

Bean, L. & D. Bean (eds) 1968. *Sir William Osler's aphorisms from his bedside teaching and writings*, 63. Springfield, IL: Charles C. Thomas.

Part I

Scientific/Historical Perspectives

Chapter 1

BSE: A Veterinary History

Lester M. Crawford

In December 1988 while appearing before a European Community (EC) parliamentary hearing in Strasbourg, France, the author received a rather earnest call from the US Embassy in London. It seemed that the Chief Veterinary Officer of the United Kingdom, Dr Keith Meldrum, was desirous of lunching at the Embassy for the purpose of discussing a matter of some urgency. Of course Meldrum was a respected member of the world veterinary and regulatory communities and had never abused his colleagueship. Dropping back by London was a bit of an imposition, but fatigue and frustration over the hormone dispute[1] in Strasbourg led to an acceptance of Dr Meldrum's offer largely because it amounted to a convenient excuse to get home a few days early. The original itinerary called for visits to several European capitals in an effort to shore up support for the US hormone position. The UK already supported the US, but perhaps the luncheon could be labeled an exercise in consolidating British support. This lame excuse perhaps prevented a later flight on Pan Am 103 (stand-by basis) five days later from London to Washington Dulles – the day of the crash over Lockerbie, Scotland.

Meldrum surprisingly brought along two colleagues to a lunch of a roast grill featuring lamb chops and beef tenderloin amongst assorted unidentifiable meats. The kitchen of the Court of St James had seen better days. The year-dated cabernet sauvignon from Ernst and Julio helped to ease the pain at least until Meldrum launched into the unappetizing subject of mad cow disease.

Following the usual battery of veterinary jokes, Keith chillingly recounted what was known about the alarming and heretofore undiagnosed disease that was sweeping through England's dairy herds.

"It's a transmissible spongiform encephalopathy, Lester," he said with uncharacteristic intensity.

"We are calling it bovine spongiform encephalopathy or BSE," whispered one of Dr Meldrum's colleagues.

"Viral, is it?" said I fighting fatigue with sharply angled phrasing. Veterinary pharmacologists, like the author, generally are bored with virology because drugs usually are ineffectual against viruses and it is the immunologist that usually solves the problem with a vaccine while pharmacologists are exhausting the research budget to no avail.

He responded, "Probably not viral in the usual sense of the word." This of course begged a further sophomoric question from the idiot American but I refrained from according my famously pompous colleagues the opening their frustrated souls longed for.

"A new disease I take it?"

Six eyes lowered like in a painting by Holbein the Younger, "Yes."

"Transmissible to humans?"

Meldrum turned the color of weathered soap stone, "Jesus, man, how can you even utter such a thing?"

"Just wondering if we should embargo British products," murmured I with a smile. No smile was returned.

The next time I saw Keith was at the World Turkey Congress in Harrogate five years later when I had left the government. He was standing beneath a giant papier mâché turkey head. After remarking about the familial resemblance, I complimented him on a job well done.

The British had indeed inherited the whirlwind. The first cases of BSE in 1986 looked every bit like rabies. But the British Isles are free of rabies, and the brains of affected cattle did not contain the negri bodies found in animals dead of rabies.

Affected cows exhibited anxiety, nervousness, and initial hyperactivity followed by lethargy. Most characteristic of the syndrome was, and is, "head-shyness". Affected animals would not allow veterinarians and others to touch their heads. Attempts to examine the horns or horn sockets or the ears were met with pronounced avoidance and obvious pain.

Post-mortem examination was unremarkable except for the consistent presence of vacuoles and astrocytic infiltration in the brain. The medulla oblongata area was spongy to the touch and microscopic examination revealed spongiform lesions or "holes" in the medullary region. The medulla contains areas that control gait, co-ordination and involuntary movements such as breathing.

These cows were suffering terribly and dying within a few days. None of them were recovering regardless of the treatment initiated. Most were older dairy cows and most were from the south of England. The British Government wasted no time in marshaling the proper expertise to analyze the situation.

Although not previously diagnosed in cattle, strikingly similar diseases had occurred in other species. Lumped under the collective term of transmissible spongiform encephalopathies (TSE), these diseases included scrapie in sheep, transmissible mink encephalopathy, and chronic wasting disease of mule deer and elk.

In humans a trio of incurable diseases – Creutzfeldt–Jakob disease (CJD), Gerstmann–Straussler–Scheinker disease and kuru – present syndromes almost too horrific to contemplate, but which nonetheless are consistent with the TSEs of the animal kingdom. The initial symptoms in people are self-neglect such as failure to groom, bathe or eat properly. This rapidly progresses to profound apathy or irritability. Sleep disorders, disorientation and tiredness may then supervene. Serious intellectual deterioration such as the inability to speak, to recognize objects, or to read and write then develop. Muscle spasms, palsies and rigid paralysis usually occur together with bizarre visual disturbances. There is no treatment. Patients usually die within one year. Most are in their late 50s at onset.

The diseases are quite rare and the incubation period can be very long – 20 years or more in humans. The shorter the natural longevity of a species, the lesser the incubation period for TSEs – cattle can be expected to develop the disease in four-and-a-half to five years, sheep somewhat less, and laboratory mice less than a year (wild mice strains which live longer may not develop the disease for two years). In humans it is of course not possible to perform experimental work, but the incubation period has been deduced from a number of cases where people were exposed to contaminated brain electrodes or contaminated pituitary extracts from cadavers only to develop CJD many years later.

Kuru presents a more astonishing story. Natives of New Guinea that engaged in a peculiar form of cannibalism, which involved eating the brains of their victims, perpetuated kuru – a typical TSE – for many years. Cessation of cannibalistic practices has abolished the disease, but not until 30 years after the last brain was eaten.

The causation of TSEs is an enigma within a mystery, and what little is known is so complex as to elude the comprehension of most people.

Early theories were that this class of diseases might be due to bacteria, viruses, or "slow viruses", an observational classification. Theorists of this persuasion were eventually disabused of these notions when it became known that normal sterilization techniques were valueless in dealing with whatever was causing this dread class of diseases. Temperatures of about 300°F sustained for an hour are required to kill the causative agent thought to be a subviral unit of some kind. It has been dubbed a "prion", a shortened form of "proteinaceaous infectious particle". Many of the hypotheses for the mode of action of the prion seem like science fiction, but most center around the prion being a glycoprotein that interacts with natural, internal brain prions to form clumps of proteinaceous material that results in the degeneration of the brain.

The British authorities could have wasted a great deal of valuable time worrying about the arcane causes of the disease. Wisely, they conducted a "down and dirty" survey to delineate what was common to the affected herds. Quickly they discovered a common link – those herds in which BSE (bovine spongiform encephalopathy) occurred had been fed offal[2] containing nervous tissues, especially spinal cords. Although not a new practice, the development of new rendering[3] procedure that used a different sterilization technique was new.

The British authorities quickly learned that those areas in England where the less intensive rendering procedure had been introduced were virtually identical to the areas where BSE was occurring. A rough hypotheses stated: the source of the infection is animal feed; therefore BSE is transmitted orally; so what we have to do is prevent the feeding of the most likely tissues, i.e. brain, spinal cord and sheep offal to cattle. These prohibitions and others were the subject of the UK's so-called "specified offal ban of 1990". The gradual decline in cases of BSE which began five years later is thought to be largely attributable to the specified offal ban.

Initially it seemed only reasonable to assume that sheep were the source of BSE since sheep had a long history of a similar disease (scrapie) and since their numbers in the UK had swelled to 44 million head because of farming subsidies. This may have been faulty reasoning; cattle cannot be infected with scrapie except by intracranial inoculation, but about 17 per cent of sheep exposed to BSE through feed contract BSE.

It is possible that BSE has existed in cattle in the UK for many years at very low levels, perhaps as low as the one new case per year per million head of cattle that would approximate the incidence of CJD in people. Indeed a case of "scrapie in an ox" was reported in 1913. The number of English cattle living long enough to manifest the disease around that time would have been approximately 1 million; one new case a year of an obscure neurological disease could have been missed.

Granted the tenuous assumption of an infinitesimal incidence, what could have happened to magnify that incidence to the 12.5 per cent experienced by 1991? Two possible factors stand out: the feeding of animal by-products (including cattle) to cattle which began slowly after the Second World War, and significant changes in the rendering process in the early 1980s. The changes were twofold: the change from batch to continuous rendering, and the elimination of solvent extraction. The first change is an unlikely suspect because the temperatures and exposure times are not dissimilar. Solvent extraction, however, is a leading suspect. Solvents such as hexane were applied to aid in the separation of the fat from the proteinaceous fractions. This also added a second high temperature step because once the fat had been separated, the solvent had to be removed by a process called steam stripping. Solvent extraction was apparently abandoned because the process produced inedible tallow that was used for candles, cosmetics, etc. Leaving the fat in the animal feed added energy to the ration, and the economics of the early 1980s augured for the shift. In the border country of northern England and in Scotland the solvent extraction process was not abandoned, and there have been very few cases of BSE.

By now, BSE has become a bovine scourge almost without parallel for a single country. Over a third of British dairy herds have been affected and the number of animals that have died number almost 200,000. New cases are still being reported because of the long incubation period.

The prohibition against using certain tissues in the production of cattle feed will, most experts agree, eventually eliminate the disease. Troublesome questions, nonetheless, remain. What is the extent of maternal transmission?[4] Is there a carrier state which could serve as a reservoir of infection? Can sheep infect cattle through other means? And, most frightening of all, can people contract the disease by drinking milk or eating beef?

This last question is presently of great concern to the British public and to other European nations, especially Germany. Sales of beef have declined by more than 20 per cent in England in the last few months of 1995 and have not fully recovered. What tipped the scales from serious interest to concern bordering on panic was the discovery in 1995 of two cases of CJD in teenagers in England, a phenomenon believed to have occurred fewer than five times in world history. The probability of finding two teenage cases in a country the size of England was infinitely small and completely unexpected and inexplicable. The rareness of the events is made the more concerning when one considers the factors that may affect the incubation period – dose, route of inoculation, inoculum strain and genetics. These young people had a shortened onset time perhaps due to an enormous exposure or to a unique mode of exposure or exposure to an unusually virulent strain.

As if to further inflame public concern, a public official opined that perhaps one of the victims had been exposed whilst inhaling feed dust containing the causative prion, a comment meant to assure all that the disease did not come from cattle or beef. To a thinking nation, as Britain certainly is, this was the worst statement that could have been made. For if the selfsame agent that is infectious to cattle is also infectious to people then beef and dairy products are by extension infectious to people.

Nineteen more human cases of a suspicious new form of CJD, by now known as v-CJD (variant-CJD) have been diagnosed. Several characteristics of the new form have convinced Britain's Spongiform Encephalopathy Advisory Committee that v-CJD is in fact a new entity probably related to BSE. All of the patients are less than 42 years old, the electroencephalogram patterns are dissimilar to that commonly seen with CJD, and the brain lesions are atypical. Even though there has not been an outpouring of new v-CJD cases, medical epidemiologists are not reassured. The worse case scenario predicts up to 85,000 British deaths.

A number of countries, including Canada, have imported English cattle that subsequently developed BSE. Much more serious is the situation in Portugal and Switzerland where BSE has become endemic; spontaneous cases are occurring in native cattle unrelated to infected UK animals or to infectious material from there. BSE now exists in Germany and France, but the source may be British cattle and/or British feedstuffs.

There have been no cases confirmed in the US, even though the US Government has had a very thorough surveillance program. Scrapie is present in US sheep and still another TSE – transmissible mink encephalopathy – is likewise present. A suspicious disease in cattle called downer cow syndrome has been investigated but appears to have no relationship to BSE. Also worrying is so-called chronic wasting disease of mule deer and elk, a TSE that has existed in the US for many years.

Much, much more research needs to be done on BSE and TSEs. But for now it appears that the British BSE epizootic is coming to an end. Transmissibility of BSE to humans remains an open question.

The great lesson of the BSE event is that the world of bacteria, viruses and prions are in a fiendish conspiracy to decimate or even extinguish higher life forms. Moreover, there is contained in the ever-evolving pool of genetic tricks available to that unseen world, the capacity to cause heretofore uncontemplated havoc to each other, to humans and to any number of non-human life forms. Thus there must be a great compunction to learn all we can from the BSE episode. The intriguing natural history of BSE might well provide a window on mechanisms of disease that may yield critical science essential to the survival of one or more species currently not at risk.

Notes

1 Between 1980 and 1989, the European Community (EC) and the US argued about the safety of meat from animals treated with certain hormones. This culminated in the EC banning US beef in 1989. The ban was lifted in 1997.
2 Although not pleasant to some, the by-products of slaughtered and dead animals are incorporated into animal feed as a convenient and cheap source of nutrition. Since such material may be an inadvertent source of infection, some experts feel safer using material from other species, like sheep by-product, for use in cattle feed.
3 Rendering is the decontamination of animal by-products by cooking at high temperatures for long periods of time with or without pressure. Obviously any modification which reduced either the time or the temperature required would be economically advantageous.
4 Recent research in England indicates that perhaps as many as 10 per cent of infected cows can transmit the infection to unborn offspring in the uterus.

Chapter 2

Transmissibility of BSE Across Species

Terri L. Harpold, Michael L. Levy and Bradley D. Savage

There is an old news adage that goes "If it bleeds, it leads", meaning simply, the story with the most graphic elements gets the most coverage. This probably had a lot to do with the intense media attention given to this story, this "epidemic" in the early 1990s, but we suggest that it had a lot to do with the "spin" put onto the story by the vegetarian or poultry lobby, to help raise the stakes and get attention. Using scare tactics and the media, the story took on a life of its own. The actual research was never reported on the six o'clock news, because prions are boring, not sexy; on the other hand, the threat of a world wide brain disease epidemic, now that could sell some papers, and the slaughtering of thousands of cows was just a bonus (as well as a reaction to the mass concern).

Every year thousands of press releases are sent to all the major news organizations, the trick is to get yours picked up and reported on. The best way to get that kind of attention is to elevate the story to one of the most basic of conditions ... fear. It worked.

Introduction

Recent reports of variant-Creutzfeld–Jakob disease (v-CJD) occurring in young UK residents has heightened the concern about the transmissibility of animal prion diseases to humans. Long before identification of a phenotypically unique human prion disease, the British legislature acted with unprecedented speed to eradicate cattle infected with bovine spongiform encephalopathy (BSE) from human and other food chains through a series of feed bans and slaughterings (Brown 1996). The World Health Organization subsequently issued even more stringent recommendations (Centers for Disease Control and Prevention 1996). Justification for the slaughter of 166,000 adult cattle over a period of seven years (Brown 1996) was founded on concern over recycling of disease-affected cattle products to healthy herds as well as possible widespread animal and human exposure to disease-affected cattle or cattle products. No experimental evidence to date has definitively demonstrated the transmissibility of BSE to humans, either by direct inoculation or through oral consumption of affected tissues. However, recent studies have identified a striking similarity in the molecular structure of BSE prion protein and prion protein from v-CJD-affected individuals. This banding pattern on Western blot differs from the characteristic pattern seen in all other classic types of CJD, raising the concern that BSE could have been transmitted to humans (Collinge et al. 1995). As the current ban on UK cattle has widespread health-related, scientific, and economic ramifications, and as the implications of BSE spread to humans are potentially devastating, this chapter will review the legislative as well as scientific events contributing to the current understanding of the BSE epidemic in the UK and will discuss chiefly the laboratory evidence which exists for the transmissibility of BSE to humans.

BSE, the Legislature, and the Public Health

In November 1986, the brains of two cattle which had suffered from unusual neurological disease were identified by the Central Veterinary Laboratory (CVL) in the UK as displaying the characteristic changes of spongiform encephalopathy. Voluntary reporting was encouraged in the 11 million cattle in Great Britain, and soon thereafter, the number of suspect cases began to rise. By December 1987, the first epidemiological studies (of some 200 affected cattle) determined that neither contact with sheep nor administration of vaccines and medicinal treatments were risk factors for subsequent development of unusual neurological disease (Collinge et al. 1995, Brown 1996). Consumption of ruminant-derived meat and bonemeal presumably containing a scrapie-like infectious agent was the only viable hypothesis for the cause of the new epidemic, which was now exceeding expected incidence rates for sporadic disease.

By June 1988, the entity known as "mad cow disease" by the public, and bovine spongiform encephalopathy by the scientific community was considered a common source epidemic and was made notifiable. Animals suspected of having BSE were restricted to the premises and isolated if about to calve in order to prevent exposure to other animals in the herd through contact with the placenta. But because spongiform encephalopathies were not considered to be contagious by simple contact, no other restriction was applied to the herd. For one month during the summer of 1988, before the Ruminant Feed Ban was enforced, restricted cattle could be removed for slaughter, though this was certainly not mandatory; the head was to be examined at the laboratory, but the remainder of tissues were permitted to be processed as any other tissue. It was not until August of that year that all suspect animals were to be compulsorily slaughtered, and their carcasses destroyed.

The Ruminant Feed Ban, enforced in July 1988, represents the key statutory measure in restricting the spread of BSE in UK cattle (Fig. 2.1) (Tyrrell & Taylor 1996). The ban specified that ruminant-derived feed (containing meat and bonemeal from potentially infected animals, notably sheep) were to be prohibited from the diet of other ruminants (notably, but not restricted to,

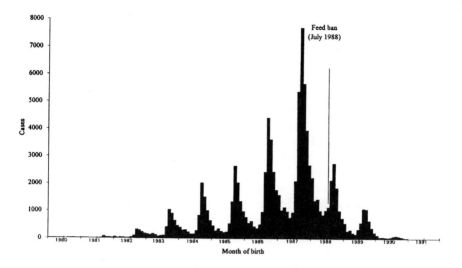

Figure 2.1 Confirmed cases of BSE with known dates of birth, plotted by month of birth (data to March 1995).

cattle). Milk, milk products, and dicalcium bone phosphate were not included in the ban.

Initial legislative efforts did not address public health, *per se*, mainly because previous experience with scrapie had not been associated with epidemiological CJD; it was assumed that BSE would likewise pose no threat to human health. Transmissibility studies, well under way, had documented transmission to mice by intracerebral inoculation, though this finding was known to be true for scrapie as well. Despite the lack of scientific evidence, the British legislature declared itself sufficiently concerned about the public's health to implement a compulsory slaughter policy for animals in whom the clinical picture was overwhelmingly one consistent with spongiform disease. The carcass was to be compulsorily destroyed. This measure, however, did not address the use and distribution of animal-derived products from cattle still in the incubation phase of these disease, and for this reason the inclusion of ruminant offal (waste) and thymus in products intended for human consumption was forbidden. The measure was known as the ban on Specified Bovine Offals (SBO).

Despite these measures, in January 1990, it was announced that five antelopes (in zoos) had succumbed to a spongiform encephalopathy. Thereafter, reports of affected great and domestic cats surfaced, with evidence suggesting strain typing of the prion protein. After the experimental transmission of BSE to pigs by simultaneous intracerebral, intravenous, and intraperitoneal inoculation, the SBO ban was extended to cover all animal species (September 1990) (Brown 1996, Collinge et al. 1996). There are no data to indicate the number of species that received the same potentially contaminated feeds as cattle, or which were

17

fed SBOs before the bans were imposed, but it is likely that far greater numbers of species were exposed who did not develop disease compared to those who did (Brown 1996).

The Spongiform Encephalopathy Advisory Committee currently considers that all the measures necessary to protect public health are now in place, including a ban on export cattle more than 30 months of age (Brown 1996, Collinge et al. 1996), and that beef produced in the UK is safe to eat. A handful of education authorities continue to ignore scientific advice and prohibit the use of British beef in school meals, despite the fact that the BSE epidemic has been on the decline since the institution of the feed ban in 1988 (Collins & Masters 1995, Brown 1996) (Fig. 2.1). The CJD Surveillance Unit produces annual reports and has had to cope with the problems of publishing information about preliminary and unreliable findings such as an apparent excess of CJD among British cattle farmers. The suggestion of such a link between BSE and CJD was rescinded after identifying a high rate of CJD in cattle farmers from European countries where BSE was rare; subsequently, CJD in cattle farmers in the UK and elsewhere was concluded to represent sporadic CJD (Collins & Masters 1995, Cousens et al. 1997).

The WHO currently recommends that no part or product of any animal that has shown signs of transmissible spongiform encephalopathy (TSE) should enter any food chain, human or animal. All countries must slaughter and prove for safe disposal of affected animals. Continuous surveillance is crucial and notification of BSE should be universally mandatory. Beef or cattle products from countries whose BSE-surveillance status is unknown should be considered unsafe. Milk and milk-products, even in countries with high incidence of BSE are considered safe. Gelatin in the food chain is considered to be safe because the manufacturing process is thought to inactivate any residual infectious activity that may have been present in source tissues. Bovine materials used for the pharmaceutical industry should only be obtained from countries with well-established surveillance protocols (Brown et al. 1994).

At the peak of the epidemic, only one in every 100 adult cattle was slaughtered as suspect. Two thirds of breeding herds have never experienced a case of BSE. Of the affected herds, 37 per cent have had only one case of BSE, and 72 per cent have had four or fewer. These figures are insignificant in terms of normal culling and replacement. $240 million has been paid already in compensation and disposal costs. British beef consumption fell by 30 per cent in 1990 following the discovery of spongiform encephalopathy in a domestic cat, but has recovered somewhat (Brown 1996). A ban on the export of British beef from cattle aged greater than 30 months persists (Collinge et al. 1996).

Variant CJD

In the spring of 1996, the British National CJD Surveillance Unit reported ten cases of CJD with a distinct clinical and neuropathological profile. Of a total 207 cases of CJD examined by the CJD Surveillance Unit (UK) between May 1990 and April 1996, ten displayed clinical and pathologic features that clearly distinguished them from the remainder. Disease onset was recent (February 1994–October 1995). Eight of the ten patients died at ages 19 to 41, with the remaining living patients aged 18 and 31 years, respectively. For the 14 years between 1970 and 1994, the total number of CJD deaths in persons less than 44 years of age were rare (total $n = 25$) and remained relatively unchanged per four year period. In 1995, however, the number of CJD deaths in the same age group rose significantly ($n = 8$), with a striking difference in the number of cases occurring in patients less than 30 years of age (Cousens et al. 1997). These cases were further distinguished from previous cases of CJD by the presence of amyloid plaques (prion protein plaques) on histopathological examination of the brain, a finding characteristic of kuru-infected brains, and one only rarely seen in cases of sporadic CJD (Diringer 1995, Cousens et al. 1997).

Although the publicity surrounding the BSE epidemic probably accounts for the improvement in case recognition of CJD in the UK in the 1990s, it remains unclear why the new variant of CJD has been seen only in young adults (Collinge et al. 1996). It was suggested that these cases represented yet another phenotype of human prion disease, separate from at least two forms of clinical presentation in "classic" CJD. Previous studies which had described distinct prion forms accounting for various strains of scrapie formed the basis for the assertion that human CJD may display strain variance as well. Because the recent cases were associated temporally and geographically, and because the new disease entity was postulated to represent a new strain of CJD, it was suggested that bovine prion protein (PrP) could have been acquired in the diets of the subjects before the SBO ban was in place; bovine PrP interacting with human PrP already present in the brain could have produced a new form of PrP^{Sc}, or prion disease (Collinge et al. 1996, Cousens et al. 1997).

Transmissibility and the "Species Barrier"

BSE is known to have caused prion disease in several other species, including domestic cats and captive exotic ungulates (nyala and kudu), presumably as a result of ingestion of BSE-contaminated feed. Transmissibility across this "species barrier" has heightened the concern that BSE may be communicable to humans. However, transgenic mice studies thus far indicate that induction of human prion production by bovine prions is inefficient (Gajdusek et al. 1996).

Transmissibility studies for spongiform encephalopathies date back to 1966 when kuru was reported to be experimentally transmissible to non-human primates by direct cerebral inoculation (Scott et al. 1989). Thirty years of experience in transmissibility studies by the same group has revealed several important findings. First, transmission rates vary for different prion diseases (100 per cent for iatrogenic CJD, 95 per cent for kuru, 95 per cent for sporadic CJD, 70 per cent for familial forms) (Collins & Masters 1995). The fact that transmission rates differ among species (10 per cent for hamsters and mice, 15 per cent for guinea pigs, and 50 per cent for cats, and 0 per cent for mink, pigs, dogs, ferrets) has suggested an empirical species barrier to passage of prion diseases.

Secondly, relative infectivity of tissue also appears to affect transmissibility. Central nervous system tissue has been consistently shown to be the most highly infectious material in animal transmissibility experiments for various prion diseases including human CJD, sheep/goat scrapie, and cattle BSE (Collins & Masters 1995). However, other tissues have been shown to be infectious, albeit at lower rates of transmissibility, and include lymph nodes, lung, liver, and kidney (Skegg 1997). The method of exposure is an additional variable in the likelihood of transmission, with direct inoculation producing the highest rates of transmission. Less direct routes, notably ingestion of infected material, are considered inefficient methods of transmission (Skegg 1997, Collins & Masters 1995).

Studies in transgenic mice support the theory of a species barrier by demonstrating that mice bearing the hamster PrP gene developed experimental scrapie (75 days after inoculation) whereas non-transgenic control mice failed to develop scrapie (> 500 days). It is hypothesized that the more dissimilar the PrP genes, the greater the species resistance to transmissibility (Collins & Masters 1995). More recent studies have focused on transgenic mice susceptible to the human prion protein disease isoform, thus providing a model for human transmissibility. To date, BSE has failed to transmit to mice lacking a species barrier to human prion disease at greater than 500 days after inoculation (Gajdusek et al. 1996). It has been postulated that differences in the primary structure of PrP molecules explains this barrier (Smith & Cousens 1996).

Strain Variance

Strain variance refers to a difference in PrP isoforms on a molecular level and is reflected characteristically in differing phenotypes of clinical disease within a given species. Strain variance in CJD had been postulated based on the strikingly different clinical courses of sporadic CJD, directly inoculated iatrogenic CJD (dura mater graft), and peripherally acquired iatrogenic CJD (human growth hormone), and has more recently been confirmed by molecular analysis (Centers for Disease Control and Prevention 1996). However, until the report of 10 cases of v-CJD, no evidence for strain variation in bovine SE had been identified (Gajdusek et al. 1966). This stands in contrast to scrapie, in which multiple natural strains have been identified, one strain of which presumably represents BSE PrP (Collinge et al. 1996, Smith & Cousens 1996).

Work by Collinge et al. (1996) has documented three distinct patterns of protease-resistant PrP banding on Western blots for sporadic and iatrogenic CJD, suggesting the presence of three distinct strains of CJD. New v-CJD can be

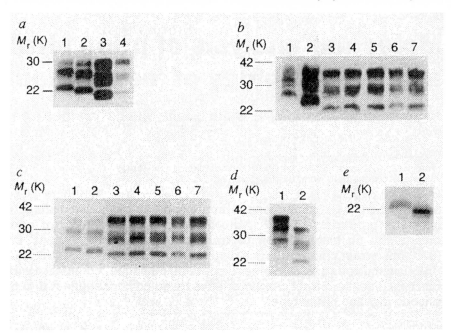

Figure 2.2 Western blots of proteinase K-treated brain homogenates from patients with sporadic and new v-CJD using anti-PrP monoclonal antibody 3F4. Numbers adjacent to horizontal bars indicate positions of M_r markers. *a*, Lane 1, type-1 sporadic CJD, *PRNP* genotype MM; lane 2, type-2 sporadic CJD, *PRNP* genotype MM; lane 3, type-3 iatrogenic CJD, *PRNP* genoptype W; lane 4, new v-CJD, *PRNP* genotype MM, "type-4" banding pattern. *b*, Lanes 1 and 2, type-1 and type-2 sporadic CJD, respectively (both with *PRNP* MM genotype; lanes 3–7, new v-CJD cases (all *PRNP* genotype MM). *c*, Lane 1, type-2 sporadic CJD, *PRNP* genotype MV; lane 2, type-2 sporadic CJD, *PRNP* genotype W; lanes 3–7, new v-CJD (all *PRNP* genotype MM). *d*, New v-CJD before (1) and after (2) treatment with proteinase K. *e*, Western blot of deglycosylated PrP. Lane 1, type-2 sporadic CJD, *PRNP* genotype MM; lane 2, new v-CJD, *PRNP* genotype MM.

clearly distinguished from all three types of CJD by a unique and highly consistent pattern of band intensities (Fig. 2.2) (Centers for Disease Control and Prevention 1996). This distinctive molecular marker, which clearly differentiates new v-CJD from sporadic CJD, serves to support the proposal, on the basis of comparative clinicopathological studies and epidemiological surveillance, that new v-CJD is a distinct and new subtype of prion disease, related to a previously unrecognized prion stain. Furthermore, when glycoform ratios and banding patterns from bovine prion protein in experimentally transmitted wild-type mice were compared with prion protein from v-CJD cases, a close resemblance was observed (Centers for Disease Control and Prevention 1996).

Discussion

There are currently eight recognized clinical disease entities affecting both humans and animals which are characterized by spongiform change upon histopathologic examination of the brain of diseased individuals. It is important to recognize that scrapie, bovine spongiform encephalopathy, kuru, Creutzfeldt–Jakob disease, Gerstmann–Straussler–Scheinker syndrome (GSS), and fatal familial insomnia are purported to have a similar, prototype molecular biological structure and mode of transmission, and as a group are best referred to as transmissible spongiform encephalopathies. That we do not conventionally refer to BSE as "cattle scrapie" as the French do reflects the original assumption that spongiform disease was primarily species-specific. Such an assumption was not initially unreasonable on empirical grounds, since clinical manifestations were initially confined to sheep (for instance) and not observed in other species.

Although sequence heterogeneity between host PrP and inoculated PrP^{Sc} was presumed to form a species barrier to transmissibility, species specificity appears to be an inconsistent finding within the TSEs. Reproducible evidence exists for the experimental transmission of many forms of TSEs to selected species, some only distantly related. On the other hand, some forms of CJD fail to transmit to mink species (and others) entirely. The issue of species impenetrability is directly challenged by the BSE epidemic itself, which is presumed to be the result of sheep PrP interaction with host bovine PrP. Such laboratory and anecdotal evidence has led some authors to assert that TSEs are eventually and invariably transmitted across species barriers (Tyrell & Taylor 1996). From such a viewpoint, v-CJD represents a phenotype of a common prion protein, and would perhaps be more accurately identified as human scrapie, or even "mad cow" disease.

Some confusion surrounds the distinction between strain variance and species variability. Multiple strains of PrP may affect any one representative of a given species and may produce distinct groupings of clinical symptoms. This stated, it is likely that some degree of transmission between species may be due to strain variance as well. In other words, although distinct strains may exist for PrP, each strain need not be species specific. Recent laboratory investigation has documented that BSE-infected material inoculated into transgenic mice produces only one strain. This strain displays the same characteristics as those found in the BSE-infected domestic cats and captive exotic ungulates (Centers for Disease Control and Prevention 1996, Collinge et al. 1996). Studies inoculating transgenic mice with v-CJD are currently underway, with results available in 1997 (Centers for Disease Control and Prevention 1996, Collinge et al. 1996).

The most striking evidence for transmissibility of BSE to humans resides in the glycoform "signature" of new v-CJD; this glycoform signature may represent a distinct strain. That this unique banding pattern (Fig. 2.2) is seen in BSE in UK cattle, in experimentally transmitted BSE in the macaque, and in naturally transmitted BSE in the domestic cat makes the argument for transmission across species more compelling. Furthermore, the likelihood that a novel, identical human PrP^{Sc} type would spontaneously occur in 12 individuals in the UK over the last two years seems extraordinarily small. The alternative conclusion, of course, is that these cases have arisen from a common source of exposure to a new prion strain.

Four more cases of v-CJD have been confirmed in the UK since March of 1996, bringing the total to 14 (Wilesmith 1996). Although this number hardly seems like an epidemic, concern has been raised that these cases may represent the beginnings of a more widespread disease, especially when the abnormally long incubation period is taken into account. For these reasons Cousens et al. (1997) have generated a mathematical model in order to provide some predictive information about where this trend will lead – and namely, how large an epidemic in humans we can expect.

The total number of new v-CJD cases predicted by the model ranges from one hundred to tens of thousands. Such a range indicates a great deal of uncertainty in the model, which would be expected based on so few established cases ($n = 14$) (Will et al. 1996). The inherent problem in the model is an inability to determine a reliable incubation period for v-CJD; Cousens selects several variable incubation period distributions for his analysis (based on kuru, for instance), which may or may not accurately reflect the incubation period for v-CJD (Wilesmith 1996).

However problematic, Cousens' study has indicated that the incidence of v-CJD in the UK cannot be adequately explained by the hypothesis that improved surveillance of the disease resulted in increased recognition of the entity. Thus v-CJD appears to be a distinct clinical entity recently emerged in Great Britain, which happens to be temporally and geographically associated with a bovine prion disease (Will et al. 1996). There is no evidence to suggest from this model that the relatively small number of cases to date assures that the resultant epidemic will also be necessarily small. Furthermore, because the incubation period is unknown, it is unlikely that cases reported over the next few years will significantly dispel much of the uncertainty surrounding the issue of proportions (Wilesmith 1996).

The biochemical evidence which exists for the structural similarity between BSE and v-CJD has been reviewed above. If further work demonstrates that v-CJD is indeed due to exposure to BSE, then the incubation period of diseases most like v-CJD (kuru and iatrogenic CJD from pituitary hormone inoculation) can be used to more definitively predict the future size of the epidemic. Establishing a more certain incubation period will also allow for a more accurate assessment of the estimated contaminated human food supply (Wilesmith 1996).

Cattle herds in the United States and in many other countries appear to be wholly unaffected and can be expected to remain so. The Centers for Disease Control and Prevention (US) reports the incidence of CJD deaths for persons aged less than 30 years at a rate of less than five cases per billion per year since

1995 (Centers for Disease Control and Prevention 1996). In Britain, the threat of continuing BSE transmission to humans has been greatly reduced, if not eliminated completely, since the feed ban took effect in 1988. Incidence rates of v-CJD will no doubt be measured closely, and if consumption of BSE-infected beef does represent a mode of transmission to humans, the incidence of v-CJD is expected to rise, though as Cousens points out, the rate of increase is indeterminable. Prior to the recent work of Collinge et al. (1996), there was no convincing evidence that v-CJD was related other than temporally and geographically to the "mad cow" epidemic; consequently, some thought the feed ban took effect prematurely. A review of the events contributing to the BSE epidemic as we have come to know it demonstrates the inherent differences in methodology for legislative and scientific processes. The initial scientific bias was necessarily against widespread legislative actions to control an epidemic no one thought was transmissible to humans. Public health officials were equally concerned with what was not yet known about transmissibility, and took action accordingly. The scientific process has now generated more than a circumstantial link between v-CJD and BSE – a structural one. In retrospect, the actions of the British legislature seem at least prudent. At present, we have a great deal to learn about the mechanism of prion propagation from one species to the next.

28 April 1997

References

Brown, P. 1996. Environmental causes of human spongiform encephalopathy. In *Prion Diseases*, H. F. Baker & R. M. Ridley (eds), 139–54. Totowa, New Jersey: Humana Press.

Brown, P., C. J. Gibbs, P. Rodgers-Johnson, D. M. Asher, M. P. Sulima, A. Bacote, L. G. Goldfarb, C. Gajdusek 1994. Human spongiform encephalopathy: the National Institutes of Health series of 300 cases of experimentally transmitted disease. *Annals of Neurology* **35**, 513–29.

Centers for Disease Control and Prevention 1996. World Health Organization Consultation on public health issues related to bovine spongiform encephalopathy and the emergence of a new variant of Creutzfeldt–Jacob disease. *JAMA* **275**, 1305–1306.

Collinge, J., M. Palmer, K. Sidle, A. Hill, I. Gowland, J. Meads, E. Asante et al. 1995. Unaltered susceptibility to BSE in transgenic mice expressing human prion protein. *Nature* **378**, 779–82.

Collinge, J., K. Sidle, J. Meads, J. Ironside, A. F. Hill 1996. Molecular analysis of prion strain variation and the aetiology of "new variant" CJD. *Nature* **383**, 685, 690.

Collins, S. J. & C. L. Masters 1995. Transmissibility of Creutzfeldt–Jacob disease and related disorders. *Science Progress* **78**, 217–27.

Cousens, S.N., E. Vynnycky, M. Zeidler, R.G. Will, P.G. Smith 1997. Predicting the CJD epidemic in humans: fourteen cases of new-variant Creutzfeldt–Jakob disease have so far been confirmed in the UK. Are they the start of an epidemic? If so, how informative will cases in the next few years be in predicting its course? *Nature* **385**, 197–8.

Diringer, H. 1995. Proposed link between transmissible spongiform encephalopathies of man and animals. *Lancet* **346**, 1208–10.

Gajdusek, D.C., C.J. Gibbs, Jr, M. Alpers 1966. Experimental transmission of a kuru-like syndrome in chimpanzees. *Nature* **209**, 794–6.

Scott, M., D. Foster, C. Mirenda 1989. Transgenic mice expressing hamster prion protein produce species-specific scrapie infectivity and amyloid plaques. *Cell* **59**, 847–57.

Skegg, D.C.G. 1997. Creutzfeldt–Jakob disease: epidemic or false alarm? *Nature* **385**, 200.

Smith, P.G. & S. Cousens 1996. Is the new variant of Creutzfeldt–Jacob disease from mad cows? *Science* **273**, 748.

Tyrrell, D.A.J. & K.C. Taylor 1996. Handling the BSE epidemic in Great Britain. In *Prion Diseases*, H.F. Baker & R.M. Ridley (eds), 175–98. Totowa, New Jersey: Humana Press.

Wilesmith, J.W. 1996. Bovine spongiform encephalopathy: methods of analyzing the epidemic in the United Kingdom. In *Prion Diseases*, H.F. Baker & R.M. Ridley (eds), 155–75. Totowa, New Jersey: Humana Press.

Will, R.G., J.W. Ironside, M. Zeidler, S.M. Cousens, K. Estibeiro, A. Alperovitch, S. Poser et al. 1996. A new variant of Creutzfeldt–Jacob disease in the UK. *Lancet* **347**, 921–5.

Chapter 3

Sheep to Cows to Man: A History of TSEs

Eve Brouwer

A Total Surprise?

In the mid-1980s, a brand new disease suddenly, and without warning, appeared among herds of British cattle.[1] The fatal malady proved to be a spongiform encephalopathy (SE) disease, so-called because of the sponge-like holes it causes in its victims' brains. Even as the disease (which most reports claimed had never before been seen among cattle) was being named bovine spongiform encephalopathy (BSE) and nicknamed mad cow disease (MCD), inferences were being made, far-reaching projections postulated, and alarms sounded in scientific circles around the world.

The inference was that scrapie, the variation of SE common to sheep, had crossed the species barrier via cattle food supplements that contain sheep carcasses. The projection was that another jump, this time from cows to people – in human food that included beef – was just as possible.

British surveillance of Creutzfeldt–Jakob disease (CJD), a variation of SE disease in humans was activated, and in early 1996 the British Government announced that there probably was a causal relationship between BSE and ten atypical cases of CJD. This prompted nearly everyone to develop an inquiring mind and demand quick, concise, simple answers to a very complicated question: was it possible that SE might have crossed yet another barrier and might be the cause of an emerging variation of one of the human forms of this disease among populations that consume beef?

A Studied but Inconclusive Past

A few research scientists stand out from among the very many who have studied and/or are continuing to study the spongiform encephalopathy (SE) diseases. Vincent Zigas, the adventurer/doctor who took the first official notice of a mysterious disease that was inexplicably spreading among his Papua New Guinea patients in 1955, brought the fatal malady – which was thought by its victims to be caused by a type of sorcery they called kuru – to the attention of other scientists; as a result, the disease was virtually eradicated and the study of

SE diseases was greatly advanced. Carleton Gajdusek was awarded a Nobel prize for his role in solving the kuru mystery. Working deep in the New Guinea jungle with Gajdusek, Michael Alpers looked beyond and through the strange, bewildering culture of the afflicted Fore tribespeople to their individual customs and focused his attention on the manner in which they prepared the bodies of their fellow tribesmen prior to burial. In so doing, he identified the incidental cannibalism, the practice of eating some of the dead tribesmen's brains, as the culprit in transmitting this particular strain of SE.

Two scientists in particular, H. B. "James" Parry and Stanley Prusiner come to center stage in this study, but don't so easily share the spotlight. Each of them has done extensive work with SE coincidentally over a 25-year period: Parry intensively tracing the origins and patterns and epidemiology of scrapie, the SE that has plagued sheep, sometimes threatened entire flocks, for at least 250 years; Prusiner doggedly searching for the agent that transmits or enables both genetic and lateral transmission of SE. These two present themselves and their findings quite differently. Where Parry appears studious, diligent, and almost conservative-to-a-fault, Prusiner seems knowledgeable, but flamboyant, somewhat self-aggrandizing and overly confident. It is a challenge to look beyond the two manners of presentation to examine their findings on their own merit. In referring to Parry's findings, words such as "proved" and "confirmed" come to mind. In referring to Prusiner's, the more questioning "claimed" and "insisted".

From Sheep to Cows?

Stanley Prusiner

For example, Prusiner, referring to "the source of the emerging epidemic", of BSE, writes and speculates that in the late 1970s, "Where once they (the processors of sheep carcasses) would have eliminated the scrapie agent in the supplement, now they *apparently* did not" (Prusiner 1995). Why "apparently"? Is he speculating? Why imply that the scrapie agent has been identified, *was* identified as long ago as the late 1970s. An irrelevant word, but it colors his credibility.

His conclusion to that paragraph steps into a near-sensationalistic mode as he notes that many people continue to worry that they will eventually fall ill as a result of having consumed tainted meat, clearly referring to the consumption of cattle and almost hinting he has reason to believe that BSE has crossed the species barrier and is posing a real threat to humans. A purely theoretical proposition could have used the human consumption of sheep: although people consume both cows and sheep, it is sheep who have suffered so heavily from an SE disease. Why not use sheep to illustrate the point? To exploit the current anxiety surrounding this topic? Because he has privileged information? Because *he* suspects that BSE is infecting humans?

Fortunately, his lapses into sensationalism are short lived, and, in the second part of his 1995 *Scientific American* article, Prusiner addresses the species barrier relative to the discovery his research team made that "the more the sequence of a scrapie PrP molecule resembles the PrP sequence of its host, the more likely it is that the host will acquire prion disease" (Prusiner 1995). But, right in the middle of explanations – of the relevancy of the ratio of divergent positions between host and recipient protein molecules, speculation that a "chaperone" protein may play a key role in helping to refold a hybrid molecule into the scrapie conformation, and/or that similarity in the central region of the PrP molecule may be the most important factor – Prusiner notes that "two farmers who had 'mad cows' in their herds have recently died of Creutzfeldt–Jakob disease" (Prusiner 1995). He proceeds to explain no further, leaving his readers to speculate on his reasons for noting this unusual "coincidence". It seems possible that the farmers, in a frugal gesture, might have butchered and eaten their diseased cows. Did they have families? Would their families not have eaten the same meat? We've heard nothing of them. Or is there an occupational hazard? Did the farmers contract the new version of CJD through contact?

H. B. "James" Parry

At the other end of the spectrum, the tone of *Scrapie disease in sheep* – a result, literally, of two writers, Parry and his editor, D. R. Oppenheimer – seems too understated at times. Speaking for himself in the preface, Oppenheimer wrote: "The idea that a disease could be at the same time hereditary and potentially infective was novel and disturbing, and seemed to involve the creation of a completely new category of disease" (Parry 1983: viii).

He was referring to the fact that Parry (whose sudden death in 1980 left his work to be finished by Oppenheimer) did not discount contagion as a cause of scrapie, but posited the controversial theory "that under natural conditions, scrapie was normally caused by an autosomal recessive gene" (Parry 1983: 94). A second controversial aspect of Parry's conviction in this regard "concerns the question of whether the postulated gene causes scrapie or whether it controls susceptibility to an infectious agent" (Parry 1983: 95). Arguing that it was unknown for susceptibility to infection to be determined by a single gene, Parry substantiated his argument that a recessive gene causes scrapie by pointing out that the infectious agent had never been found in non-affected animals (Parry 1983: 95).

A Human Connection?

In 1978, in the letter accompanying submission of his genetic study, "Natural scrapie in sheep: its natural history and disappearance following genetic procedures" (a study that Oppenheimer viewed as producing "seemingly incontrovertible evidence that there is a single gene which controls" the inherited occurrence of scrapie (Parry 1983: 95)), Parry wrote: "In view of the wide interest aroused in the general subject of the Transmissible ('Slow Virus') Dementias of Man and Animals by Dr. Gajdusek's Nobel Prize Oration last year, it seems important to place on record facts regarding scrapie in sheep which are generally overlooked in the scramble to establish a primary infectious etiology for this group of disorders" (Parry 1983: Appendix A, 159).

Parry's warning was placed "on record". The article was accepted and published (Parry 1983: Appendix A, 159). Nonetheless, it appears that Parry's call for caution went virtually unheard and had no influence on the allegedly common practice of enriching cattle feed by adding sheep waste to it. On the contrary, shortly after Parry wrote the above, the animal feed industry allegedly began phasing out the use of hydrocarbon solvents and high temperatures in rendering animal remnants (Watts 1996), a change that is now held responsible – accurately or not – for the apparent transmission of SE from sheep to cattle.

Parry's area of study focused narrowly and intensely on the sheep industry, but he did continue in the same letter with a broader warning: "The implications of these results are also important for the policies of Government, Veterinary, and Agricultural Departments around the world, who view scrapie, quite properly, as a very serious matter" (Parry 1979; ibid. 1983: Appendix A, 159).

Adding weight to his claim that this is a serious matter, in his book, *Scrapie disease in sheep*, Parry draws attention to a society of Jews in Libya who, finding sheep eyes and brains a tasty delicacy, regularly consume them ... and also experience a 30-fold increase in the incidence of CJD compared to the rest of the world. Regardless of this striking correlation, Parry concludes that because he has not studied the rate of CJD among other ethnic groups in the region who also eat eyeballs and brains of sheep, he cannot draw a conclusion as to a cause and effect relationship between consumption of these parts of the sheep and CJD (Parry 1983: 148). Parry wrote, in regard to danger of transmission of SEs from sheep to humans, "Its alleged connection with human disease[2] rests on presumptions for which satisfactory evidence is lacking" (Parry 1983: Appendix A, 168).

In regard to handling and working with SE diseased sheep, primarily referring to his 31 years of observing shepherds, owners, slaughtermen, and butchers for signs of CJD or a variation thereof, Parry concluded that scrapie presents no occupational hazards. But Prusiner's references to the two farmers who died of CJD following the deaths of their mad cows, re-ignites questions as to whether there is a correlation between the two or if an occupational hazard exists.

Of course, Parry and Prusiner are not the only ones to bring attention to this point: if John Darnton's report in the 21 March 1996 *New York Times* is correct when he writes that four victims in the first group of ten people diagnosed with the new strain of CJD are dairy farmers, "some whose herds had been infected with bovine spongiform encephalopathy", it would seem that such extremely disproportionate statistics indicate a need to continue to explore the possibility that handling live animals suffering from an SE may pose an occupational hazard. This is contrary to the assurances of the Advisory Committee on Dangerous Pathogens and Department of Health's 1994 bulletin that "There is no evidence to suggest that close contact with TSE-infected animals presents an infection risk and no special precautions are required when handling an intact diseased animal."

Parry said he could genetically control and eradicate SE in sheep because the disease is caused by a single recessive gene. Prusiner says prions are responsible. Prion is the name given by Prusiner for the mutant form of PrP, a common-to-all-life protein. According to Prusiner, prions can inexplicably and randomly trigger the domino effect, which is characteristic of SE, involving the refolding and subsequent malformation of other proteins with which it comes in contact. These prions "can also cause sporadic disease, in which neither transmission between individuals nor inheritance is evident" (Prusiner 1995).

The Kuru Questions

That Vincent Zigas, in *Laughing death, the untold story of kuru,* clearly intended to set the record straight in regard to personal and political issues is clear from the book's foreword, written by Carleton Gajdusek after Zigas's death, and seems more a disclaimer than the typical glowing accolade that one would expect. Zigas's determination to emphasize his own altruistic intentions – as well as to analyze, invariably with less generosity, the personalities and motivations of all the other scientists who became involved in the study – ironically lends credibility to the account. While his attempt at page-turning prose is unsuccessful, his approach to kuru is interesting, especially because it raises some unusual questions.

The pattern that kuru followed as it worked its way through the Fore may be relevant to the current concern. Is the SE incubation period shortened if ingestion is the method of transmittal? And/or is the chance of transmittal increased if the disease is clinically active? Today's concerns don't focus on whether ingestion is a feasible method of transmission but, rather, on the issue of whether the species barrier was inadvertently bridged.

Of course, almost all of today's factors are different from the kuru situation; but one similarity, the early age of onset, invites comparison. According to Zigas, many Fore children contracted kuru, raising the question of why the incubation period was so greatly reduced.

A plausible scenario might have been that the kuru cycle began with a one-in-a-million case of CJD that occurred naturally among the Fore tribe and was then transmitted latterly via ingestion. Unfortunately, as the (usually) women performed the customary burial preparations – suctioning the brain from the dead person's skull, licking the straw as they worked, sharing it with their children – they put themselves and the children in jeopardy, and in a few years the signs were evident that the disease had been transmitted to both the women and the children, and that they, as secondary hosts, had contracted the disease. Then, when they died and their bodies were likewise prepared for burial, the disease was passed on yet again to tertiary hosts who quickly exhibited signs of disease and died. As Zigas tells the story, the cycle apparently accelerated as it continued; the incubation periods seemed to grow progressively shorter; and the disease attacked victims at atypically younger and younger ages.

That the disease definitely was clinically active before the Fore ingested the transmittal agent invites another question. Is the disease more easily transmitted if it has manifested itself clinically in the host? Were the Fore at increased risk because they ingested matter from causalities of clinically-active SE?

These questions of whether the incubation periods are shorter in secondary hosts, and whether the possibility of transmission is increased if SE is clinically active, touch on areas that contribute to the current panic regarding human consumption of "mad" cows. Even though sheep also are consumed by humans and have, in fact, a much longer history of SE disease, cows might be more likely to be eaten when they're old enough to have a clinically-active SE disease. With the exception of the Libyan Jews cited earlier, people generally eat sheep when they are still lambs. The lambs may be genetic carriers of SE, but, as the primary hosts, they're too young for the disease to have become clinically active.

The Heat Factor

Another substantive point to consider in exploring this issue is the relationship between the cooking of infected tissue and its potential for infectivity. Documented cases of infective matter (kuru and transplants) are uncooked tissue. If it is true that lowering the temperature was one of the crucial changes made in the process of rendering animal remnants for cattle feed in the late 1970s, it would seem that a barrier against transmittal was weakened.

Insofar as the heat factor applies directly to humans, people generally cook lamb more thoroughly than they do beef. If heat inactivates the PrP, the popularity of steak tartar and raw or nearly raw beef dishes (contrasted, on the other hand, to the traditional ways of cooking lamb), might contribute to the possibility that BSE poses a threat to humans.

Another Barrier

In fact, if the disease did manage to cross the species barrier – as other diseases such as brucellosis, *Escherichia colians, salmonella* infection, and bovine tuberculosis (Lappe & Bailey 1996) have – and if it were transmitted from sheep to cows, it might indeed, as with the secondary hosts who contracted kuru, need a shorter incubation period before becoming clinically active in the cattle. Following that line of thought, once it became clinically active in its relatively young secondary hosts, these beef cows could hold the same threat to the human population as the sheep had held for – and apparently delivered to – the cattle. With one more crossing of the species barrier, a new strain of SE, one with yet a shorter incubation period could be transmitted to humans.

Some might believe that the government agencies that inspect food sources and remove questionable products from the food chain, stand at the ready, poised to guard most of the civilized world from attacks of this kind. But even if these government agencies were operating at optimal performance, early symptoms of the disease are slight and extremely difficult to detect. Veterinarian Dr William Hueston, speaking on behalf of the US Department of Agriculture's (USDA) Animal and Plant Health Inspection Service (APHIS), optimistically says, "The federal government, cattle industry, and food manufacturers are working together to ensure a safe food supply for the American consumer. They have effective inspection programs and monitoring systems in place to ensure that beef and food or consumer products derived from cattle are safe to eat and do not contain BSE" (Food Insight 1996). Less optimistically, writers Marc Lappe and Britt Bailey (1996) contend that American beef-eaters are in this respect "terribly vulnerable" because USDA inspection of a beef carcass cannot pick up subtle clues of neurodegeneration, and the surveillance system the USDA uses to monitor potential BSE cases only picks up overtly sick BSE-infected cattle.

But if these monitoring agencies are stringent enough to be able to discern whether or not cows are suffering from early stages of SE is beside the point. In addition, other equally insubstantial topics serve as smokescreens that divert attention rather than address the issues. For example, the media was heard to proclaim on US newscasts that although British cows have been imported, there is no evidence they have infected American cows. In another newscast, farmers said they thought it was "perverse" to feed meat to herbivores and claimed they wouldn't have done it if the cattle feed had been labeled. This complaint is particularly interesting in light of the many cattle breeding practices – such as branding, castration, artificial insemination and so forth – that also seem so overtly perverse.

Protecting the Common Good

In fact, these and other similarly pointless arguments merely serve to cloud the relevant facts:

(a) in kuru we had a vivid picture of how easily SE disease can move among a population;
(b) at the least, Parry proved that SE disease can be controlled through genetic selection;
(c) finally, it certainly is possible for disease to cross species barriers.

If a new variation of CJD is "emerging", as it may very well be, it will affect (kill) people. Fortunately, unlike kuru, it will not be passed among its tertiary hosts (because they do not consume each other upon death), but will die out as its victims die.

As other theories are formulated, more questions arise. One unusual theory raises many questions in suggesting that all CJD cases are due to transmission from animals to human beings (Diringer 1995). Estimates attributing only 5 to 15 per cent of CJD cases to genetic sources imply that the remaining 85 to 95 per cent of unexplained cases are caused iatrogenically, through corneal transplants, dura mater grafts, and intravenously-administered growth hormone derived from pooled human pituitary glands. In another interesting study, similar findings resulted from comparisons made between British farmers who suffered from atypical CJD and French, German and Italian farmers who were likewise afflicted, allowing the possibility that the British cases were no more related to BSE than the continental cases were (Gore 1996).

Conclusion

At the least, it would be prudent to do everything possible to remove SE from the food sources perhaps by:

(a) finding and recommending cooking practices that inactivate the PrP;
(b) genetically controlled breeding of sheep to remove scrapie from flocks that are going to be fed to cows;
(c) stopping the practice of using sheep (and/or other ruminants) in animal feed;
(d) changing the way in which sheep are processed for feed so that the transmissible SE agent is not included in the feed;
(e) removing infected cows from the human food chain.

If these measures are not enacted, many more instances of the new strain of spongiform encephalopathy disease will probably follow these 15 very well-publicized cases.

Notes

1 Dr Lauren Mets, Associate Professor, Department of Molecular Genetics and Cell Biology, of the University of Chicago, was extremely helpful to me as I researched spongiform encephalopathies. I greatly appreciated his support. Dr Mets cannot, however, be held responsible for the content herein; the arguments and conclusion are mine.
2 As his source, Parry refers here to D. C. Gajdusek "Unconventional viruses and the origin and disappearance of Kuru", *Science* **197**, 943–60.

References

Advisory Committee on Dangerous Pathogens 1994. *Precautions for work with human and animal transmissible spongiform encephalopathies.* London: HMSO.

Advisory Committee on Dangerous Pathogens and Department of Health 1996. *Precautions for work with human and animal transmissible spongiform encephalopathies.* Bulletin, 18 April. HSE Information Centre, Sheffield.

Diringer, H. 1995. Proposed link between transmissible spongiform encephalopathies of men and animals. *The Lancet* **346**, 1208–10.

Food Insight 1996. The beef about BSE and US food safety. International Food Information Council Foundation, Washington, DC.

Gore, S.M. 1996. More than happenstance: Creutzfeldt–Jakob disease in farmers and young adults. *British Medical Journal* **311**, 1416–19.

Lappe, M. & B. Bailey 1996. Mad about beef. *Chicago Tribune* 25 April.

New York Times, 1-12-96, John Darnton, Fear of mad-cow disease spoils Britain's appetite.

Parry, H.B. 1983. *Scrapie disease in sheep.* London: Academic Press.

Prusiner, S.B. 1995. The prion diseases. *Scientific American* **272**, 48–57.

Watts, M. 1996. Turning cows into cannibals. *Independent* 31 March.

Zigas, V. 1990. *Laughing death, the untold story of kuru.* New Jersey: Humana Press.

Chapter 4

Can the Spread of BSE and CJD be Predicted?

Steven Dealler

The epidemic of BSE (bovine spongiform encephalopathy) in the UK can be analyzed using various methods and statistical models. To decide which is the right one requires a knowledge of the disease itself, how it multiplies, and how it is passed from one animal to another. Initial mathematics require simply an analysis of the Gaussian curve produced from results correlated by the Ministry of Agriculture, Fisheries and Food (MAFF) in the UK (MAFF 1996a, b). However, such mathematical models cannot adequately predict the future of the disease, but alternative methods, which take into account the biology of the disease, can be used to give a better indication.

I will discuss the biology of this type of disease and the models of the BSE epidemic that have been considered, examine the data on case numbers available from MAFF, and then describe how these figures can be used to give some idea of the human and bovine risks.

BSE as One of the TSES

BSE is one of the transmissible spongiform encephalopathies (TSES). TSES are fatal, with no method of diagnosis before death or treatment. It is a slowly developing illness in which the agent appears to pass from peripheral tissues to the central nervous system and to cause pathology through the production of highly resistant proteinaceous prions (PrPres). These are derived from a normal protein, the prion protein (PrPc), that is carried on the surface of many cellular groups, particularly nerves, lymphocytes, and macrophages. Of these it is the nerves that do not continuously multiply and so the amount of PrPres builds up in association with them, eventually causing neuronal damage.

TSE infectivity has been found in almost all the tissues of the body, but it is much higher in the brain than elsewhere (Dealler 1993). Infectivity can be detected by inoculating tissue into the brain of another animal of the same species. The technique is much less sensitive if a different species is used for the test; for instance, inoculating mice with tissue from cattle with BSE produces a 1000-fold fall in infectivity; but the tissues cannot be considered to be non-infectious just because the mouse does not develop disease. This "species-barrier" effect is dependent not only on the species but also on strains within the species. As it happens, however, cattle in the UK appear to be of a similar strain. When crossing this barrier the disease has a relatively long incubation period in the recipient animal, with histopathological changes that are abnormal and unreliable. However, when passed on again from the recipient animal to another of the same species, the incubation period of the disease drops and the pathology becomes regular and reliable.

There appears to be *strains* of TSE infection, although that has not been shown for BSE. A different strain will produce a separate incubation period, a set of specific symptoms before death, and recognizable histopathology.

The *dose* that is required to transmit a TSE does not act in the same way as a virus; the number of infectious particles required to pass the disease by mouth is around 10^4–10^5 times that needed by inoculation into the CSF (the amount is known as 1 infectious unit, IU); 9 IU into the blood have been shown to be adequate to cause infection. Also, the dose alters the incubation period; larger doses give shorter incubation periods. This is reliable enough to be used to measure the levels of infectivity present in specific tissues by doing a test inoculation into an animal and then measuring its incubation period. Brain tissue of a cow with clinical BSE has been shown to have approximately 10^5 IU per gram when inoculated into a mouse. When inoculated into a cow it would

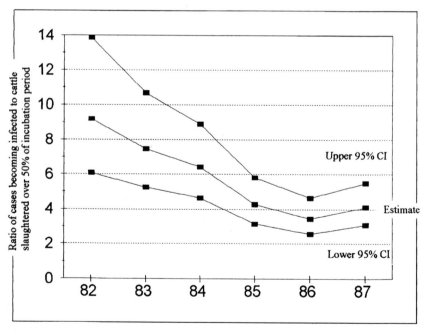

Figure 4.1 R values, or ratio of animals providing infection to those becoming infected (data as calculated from MAFF figures taking underreporting into account).

Table 4.1a Animals known to have become infected with spongiform encephalopathy epidemiologically related to BSE

Species	Date of first report
Nyala	1986
Gemsbok	1987
Arabian oryx	1989
Greater kudu	1989
Eland	1989
Domestic cat	1989
Moufflon	1989
Ostrich (yet to be confirmed as being associated with BSE)	<1991
Puma	1991
Cheetah	1992
Scimitar horned oryx	1993
Ocelot	1994
Tiger	1995
Rhesus monkey	1996
Macaque monkey	1996
Ankole cow	1996
Human (to be confirmed)	1996
Bison	1997

be expected to contain 10^8 IU per gram. The brain of a cow weighs 250 g and would be expected to contain 2.5×10^{10} IU, i.e. enough, by oral feeding, to carry the disease to around 2.5×10^5 other cattle. However, the transmission rate was much lower than this (Fig. 4.1).

Although certain strains appear to be immune naturally to certain TSEs, no acquired immunity seems to take place and this may be why some groups feel that a cumulative infection is present. BSE is already thought to have infected 24

Table 4.1b Species susceptible to BSE following experimental challenge

Species	Year of report	Intracerebral inoculum	Oral inoculum
Cattle	1989	+ve	+ve
Mouse	1988	+ve	+ve
Sheep	Challenged in 1988	+ve	+ve
Goat	Challenged in 1988	+ve	+ve
Marmoset monkey	1990	+ve	Not tested
Pig	1991	+ve	In progress
Mink	1994	+ve	+ve

species (Tables 4.1a, b), but there must be some that have been exposed to an infectious agent (as they have been fed the same material) and yet not developed disease (domestic dogs).

Biological Models of Disease

An initial model (Model 4.1) was designed to explain how BSE infected many cattle and spread without a specific known source. It soon became clear that such a model could not explain the whole story. Sheep and cattle had been living together for many years in the UK and yet no cases of BSE had been previously reported. The first cases of BSE that were seen did not have a particularly long incubation period. Indeed there seems statistically to have been no drop in the incubation period (as should have taken place if the disease came from sheep). The distribution of histopathology produced by BSE in a test mouse was different from that produced by six strains of scrapie (Foster et al. 1996). All that could be suggested was that perhaps the cattle that derived BSE from sheep did so much earlier on and so we did not see those cases. In the USA, rendered offal meal, although used in smaller quantities as feed for cattle, has been produced in the same manner and yet no outbreak of BSE has occurred. Several self-sufficient UK farmers, who do not buy any manufactured feed and breed all replacement stock have had cattle with BSE. Cases of BSE have appeared in cattle (in large numbers) since the ban in offal meal took place in June 1988.

One of the major problems was that meal arrived on a farm in batches and some batches would be expected to contain infected material and others would not. As the epidemic progressed it was assumed that, for any one calf the time it

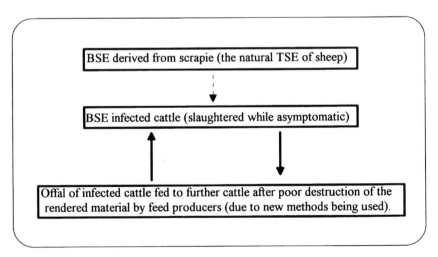

Model 4.1

would be expected to wait before being exposed to a dangerous batch would get shorter and so the time between birth and symptoms would shorten. This was not seen, although pains were taken to look for the phenomenon. A minor drop in this period was found but was felt to be explained by the farmers and veterinary officers becoming more experienced in recognizing cases and could do so earlier in the symptomatic period. No association could be found between the use of specific feeds with disease, and the infecting agent has never been found in bovine meal.

The number of cases that appeared in the UK and the number of calves with BSE born after the feed ban in 1988, has risen to represent around 50 per cent of the cattle seen with disease at the current time (Owen 1996). Attempts have been made to see if any specific cause for this is present. Initially it was felt that it was entirely due to infective material getting into feed or the cattle being fed pig meal, which was still produced using bovine rendered products until 1994. One study looked at 315 cattle from dams infected with BSE and 315 controls from dams that had died by the age of six years without BSE. It was found that 19 control and 47 test offspring developed BSE, a vertical transmission rate of 10 per cent (95% confidence interval (CI): 5%–15%). It did not explain how the 19 per cent became infected (Spongiform Encephalopathy Advisory Committee 1996).

A new model (Model 4.2) was produced. A problem has appeared with this model in that only a certain proportion of the cattle in a herd appear to become infected. The in-herd infection rate has risen to around 2.5 per cent per annum but gone little higher. Logically, as the case numbers rose, the amount of infective material present in the feed should have risen in parallel to this, and

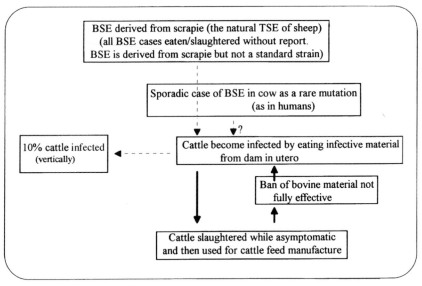

Model 4.2

the number of cattle becoming infected should have risen as well. To explain the low in-herd rate of BSE, it was suggested that those cattle with disease were the only ones that *could* be infected for some genetic reason. When this was tested by looking at the prion protein gene of BSE cases and controls, no difference was found between the two groups (Curnow et al. 1993).

Scrapie inoculated into mice produced the disease, but with a different distribution of brain tissue histopathology than BSE (Foster et al. 1996). Scrapie when inoculated into cattle did not produce BSE, which also seemed to infect a different range of animals. No expected incubation period drop could be seen following transmission from sheep. Originally BSE would have appeared in 1979–80 (had we known to look), but the changes in the meat and bonemeal manufacturing procedures have been taking place since 1972. If BSE was derived from scrapie, which had been present throughout the period, the epidemic would surely have been expected to start earlier. BSE-infected bonemeal was also fed back to sheep, and no increase in scrapie has been adequately reported. The report from the USA of transmissible mink encephalopathy in a mink ranch fed with only beef meat suggests that BSE is a rare sporadic disease (Marsh 1990).

Following these findings further alterations were required to produce Model 4.3. The apparent 'window effect' has, however, never been noticed adequately in other species; an apparently similar one is seen in sheep (in that they develop scrapie between two and four years and no later), but no investigation has taken place. The exact cause of it is unclear as no immunity is known to develop to a TSE. What this model also unexplained is the low in-herd rate (Table 4.2) and the reason that it does not rise in parallel with the national

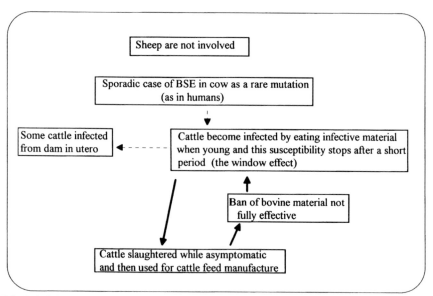

Model 4.3

Table 4.2 Number of cattle with BSE reported has apparently declined

Year	No. of cattle	Year	No. of cattle
1987	7	1992	36681
1988	2184	1993	34370
1989	7136	1994	23944
1990	14181	1995	14076
1991	25027	1996	7202

rate. After all, if the infection appears randomly in bags of meal it would be as if a cow had randomly won a lottery ticket and the more tickets there were, the more winners. What has actually happened is that the in-herd rate has remained stationary and in order to have an epidemic it has been the number of affected herds that has actually risen (see Appendix 2).

Various models permit the epidemiology that is seen; the most favoured is shown in Model 4.4.

This model fulfils the known epidemiological problems; it is the offspring of the meal infected cow that we see with the disease, not the cow that ate the infected material itself. The major problem with this is the possibility it brings

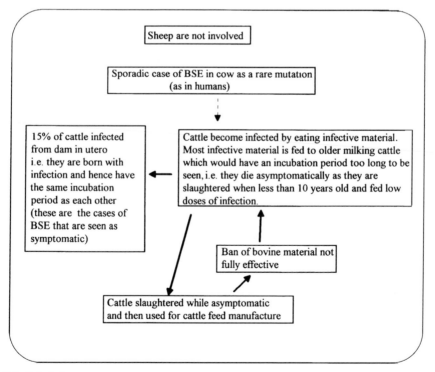

Model 4.4

forward that a very large proportion of the dairy cattle in the UK became infected from feed, e.g. 60 per cent to 90 per cent leading up to the peak in 1988; however, this is the sort of percentage that is found in other TSEs so we must not avoid this because it is a politically undesirable finding. It would explain why the rate of BSE in cattle born after that date fell so slowly and in parallel with the drop in infected dams that took place owing to slaughter at the end of their milking lives. It would also explain why such a low proportion of cattle in affected herds showed any symptoms. Some herds, however, have had much higher proportions of cattle that are affected; perhaps there is a further factor that is involved; environmental contamination with prion-type agents must be considered because 99.9 per cent of infection is thought to pass through into the feces and remain infective. As such, are further models (Model 4.5) now needed?

Mathematical modeling, however exact, has great difficulty in working out the size of these compartments as the information available from MAFF is purely that of the percentage of infected offspring; there is little opportunity to work out what is happening elsewhere.

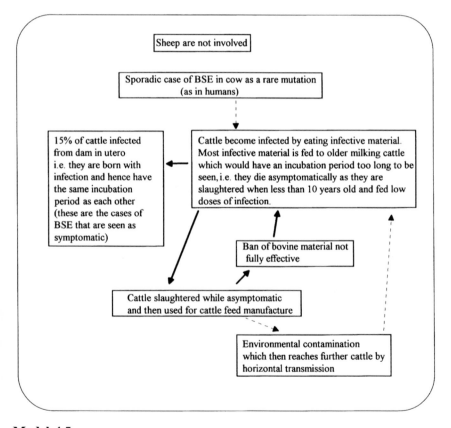

Model 4.5

Mathematical Data for the Cases of BSE in the UK

Information for this is derived from MAFF statistics (after great difficulty in getting its release (Editorial, *Nature* 1996)) but there are difficulties in the interpretation of MAFF data. The reported number of cases of BSE that have been put under restriction, slaughtered, and then confirmed by histology are shown in Table 4.2. Perhaps a better indicator of the way in which the epidemic has progressed can be seen from Figure 4.2 as this also shows the way in which political pressure, knowledge of disease, and compensation levels have possibly altered the number of cases that have been reported.

An attempt was made to assess the level of underreporting by accepting the reporting of two years – 1990 and 1991 – as being reasonably valid. The reason for this was that farmers were at that time seeing few cattle and the level of compensation was relatively high compared to the absolute value of the animal. Little advantage was seen to not admitting a case except a social one amongst the farmer's peers. When the results for cases born after the feed ban and reported in 1992 and 1993 are corrected for the size of the population that had succumbed to BSE from that group in 1990 and 1991 it is seen that the underreporting is unacceptably high (Table 4.3). True case numbers from the years following 1993 are more difficult to calculate and later work has not attempted to estimate underreporting (Anderson et al. 1996).

Initially it was expected that the number of cases of BSE in cattle born after the feed ban would be very low, if not zero by some. The series of graphs shown in Figure 4.2 shows how it is possible to initially convince oneself that things are getting better. However, it is necessary to calculate not just the number of cases that you can see but, in order to compare years, it is necessary to find the number that will die by a certain age. When this is carried out using the data from Table 4.2 and the age/case proportion graph of Table 4.5 it can be seen that following the feed ban there was not as great a fall in cases as was expected; statistically, no effect was seen by 1993 (Figure 4.3).

The method of calculation of underreporting becomes less valid in later years as the numbers of cattle are less related to those in 1990–91. There has, however, been no attempt to produce data indicating true rates rather than

Table 4.3 Estimated percentage of BSE cases reported to MAFF using statistical assessment

	Reporting year			
	1992		1993	
Year of birth	Estimate	95% CI	Estimate	95% CI
1987–8	78	70–87	66	58–74
After 1987–8	53	32–87	39	24–65

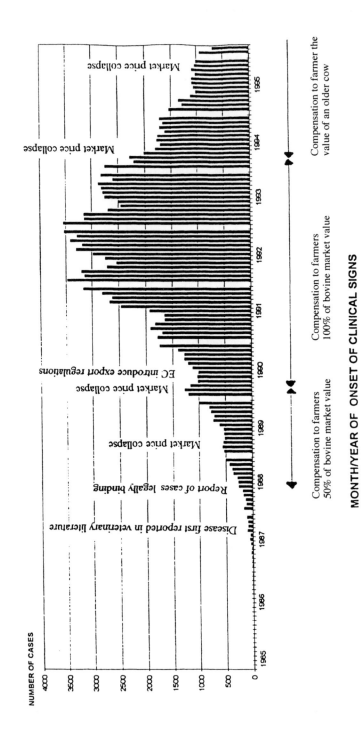

Figure 4.2 Number of cases with onset of clinical signs in specific months.

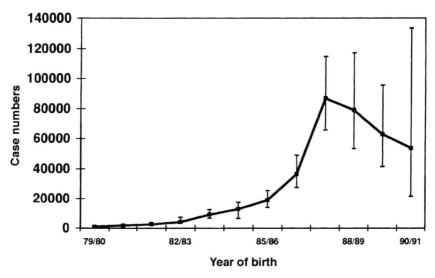

Figure 4.3   Annual BSE incidence following corrections for underreporting.

apparent rates of disease and the recent predictions (Table 4.4) of Anderson et al. (1996) assumed that all cases were reported and diagnosed.

The results given above concerning vertical transmission were simply those released by the Spongiform Encephalopathy Advisory Committee at the beginning of August 1996. Anderson's calculations were carried out using the standard Model 4.3 and attempting to indicate that a 10 per cent vertical transmission rate in the last six months of the incubation period of the mother would the BSE rate as seen in UK farms, particularly in 1995. It is not, however, made clear how this is justified as, whatever the rate of vertical transmission, exactly the same rate of disease could have been produced by those cattle eating excess infective meal. Indeed, Models 4.4 and 4.5 could also be valid and fit the epidemiology that is seen.

Table 4.4   Predicted statistics of Anderson et al. (1996) for the epidemic of BSE in the UK assuming that 10 per cent maternal transmission takes place in the last six months of BSE incubation in a dam

Year	No. of maternal transmissions	95% CI	No. of BSE cases expected to be reported	95% CI
1996	189	155–11300	7386	6541–8856
1997	95	63–236	4111	3006–7664
1998	38	21–214	1864	1152–7025
1999	12	5–162	682	388–5909
2000	3	1–86	221	128–3660
2001	1	0–33	72	45–1592

Table 4.5   Proportion of the cattle that die of BSE during each year of age

Age (years)	Proportion	95% CI range
2	0.0016	0.0008–0.0024
3	0.048	0.043–0.053
4	0.239	0.224–0.255
5	0.304	0.295–0.313
6	0.209	0.202–0.217
7	0.101	0.093–0.109
8	0.047	0.041–0.054
9	0.029	0.023–0.035
10	0.018	0.013–0.024

It came as a surprise when many of the cattle that developed BSE were born after the feed ban of 1988. Initially this was thought to be due to bags of infective meat and bonemeal not having been disposed of, then arguments were put forward that it was bovine tallow present in it that transmitted the disease, then it was suggested that pig meal was being fed to cattle. However, all of these suggestions would not be adequate to explain the minor change that was seen in BSE for cattle born before and after the feed ban. It can be seen from Figure 4.4 that many of the cattle developing BSE were born in an extended period after the ban and when, using the data from Table 4.4, these figures are corrected to calculate the number of cases that would be seen by the age of ten years in each of the groups, it can be seen that the epidemic will be expected to continue after the year 2000 (data not shown).

Human Risk

Initially no data was available for the number of cases of cattle infected with BSE that were eaten by the human population. This was, however, calculable by correcting the case numbers of BSE according to the age distribution for the cattle seen in the UK bovine population (Dealler 1993, Dealler & Kent 1995, Anderson et al. 1996). When this is done the number of infected cattle shown to have been eaten has been reported in several ways; Anderson et al. (1996) claimed that we would have eaten 446,000 (95 per cent CI, 440,000–580,000) infected cattle by the start of the specified bovine offal ban in 1989 and between then and the end of 1995 a further 283,000 (95 per cent CI; 270,000–330,000). These results did not take into account the underreporting of cases that was taking place in the UK since 1992. Dealler & Kent (1995) calculated that the number eaten would be 1.8 million (95 per cent CI, 1.1 million–3.2 million) before 2001, but this did take into account the apparent underreporting that took place. Without allowing for underreporting a previous calculation, Dealler showed 1.1 million to be a closer approximation (data not shown).

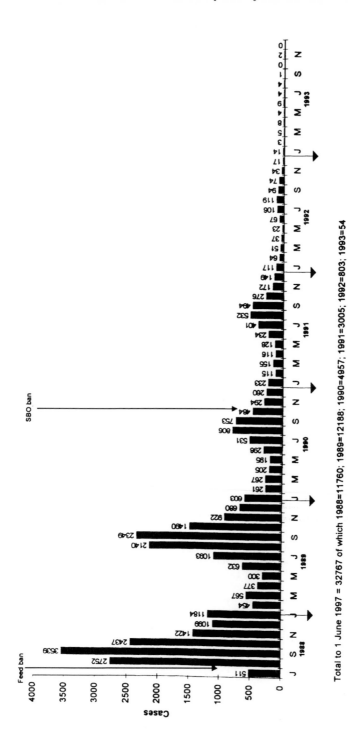

Figure 4.4 BSE confirmed in cattle born after 18 July 1988; total to 1 June 1997 (derived from the Ministry of Agriculture, Fisheries and Food document, *Bovine Spongiform Encephalopathy in Great Britain. A progress report June 1997*).

47

Attempts to assess the risk that has been taken by the human population has been done in two ways. Dealler & Kent (1995) assumed that the level of infectivity present in bovine tissue to be similar to that found in the tissues of other animals with TSE. When this is done it is possible to estimate the total amounts of infectivity entering the human food chain but the possible range is found to be wide with 13 out of 21 figures for the potential number of people becoming infected being over 100,000 and 11 being in millions. However eight of the figures were zero. What can be said is that when the same statistical estimation was done for scrapie, only two of the figures were not zero and the doses of infectivity present in the human diet were expected to be 10,000 to 100,000 times higher with BSE than with scrapie. A second method by Dealler depends on the number of people that would have become infected at different points in the epidemic (Dealler 1996). It assumes that the cases of variant CJD seen already were infected at the same point in the epidemic. At whatever point

Table 4.6 Case numbers of BSE in humans (as variant CJD) as predicted by Dealler (1996)

Year	Number of cattle eaten by the human population in specific years at 50% or greater of incubation period	Total number of people expected to die of CJD assuming that the 10 cases represent specific percentages of those infected in this, the first year of infection			
		100%	10%	1%	0.1%
1982	274	2141	21440	214100	2141000
1983	675	617	6170	61700	617000
1984	1415	248	2480	24800	248000
1985	3012	109	1090	10900	109000
1986	5510	54	540	5400	54000
1987	8908	30	300	3000	30000
1988	14279	17	170	1700	17000
1989	24606	10	100	1000	10000

These figures assume that nobody ever became infected with BSE after the Specified Offals Ban was introduced in November 1989. Also assumed is that all cattle with symptomatic BSE in 1990 and 1991 were recognized by farmers, reported by them, accepted by veterinary officers, slaughtered, and correctly diagnosed by neurohistology. Little difference is, however, seen in these figures if the proportion of total cases that reaches MAFF statistics remains steady throughout the epidemic.

In order to understand this table it is necessary to decide which year the ten people became infected in and what proportion of the people infected in that year is represented by the ten people. As such the total number of people expected to become infected lies between 10 and 2,141,000.

Using a different technique, a range of 99–80,000 cases has been predicted, depending on the incubation period of the disease, but the authors admit that the accuracy of this could be depressingly low (Cousens 1997).

that was we could calculate the number of infected cattle that had been eaten by that time in order to cause these cases and so predict the number that would appear as a result of people eating larger numbers later in the epidemic (Table 4.6). The only help in indicating which of the figures in Table 4.6 would be the right one would be indicated by estimates as to what would be expected to be the incubation period (ip) for BSE in humans. This depends on the ip of TSE being related to the normal life expectancy of the animal – it is generally around 10 per cent to 15 per cent when a large dose of inoculum is used. When crossing from another species, however this ip is often double this and, when a small dose is used for transmission, the ip is higher again. These would merely suggest that BSE in humans might be expected to have a very long ip; possibly over 20 years. As such, it would suggest that the figures towards the top of Table 4.6 were most significant and that between 2000 and 2,000,000 would seem reasonable. Neither of these methods are satisfactory but it is unlikely that we will get more exact predictive figures for several years.

References

Anderson, R. M., C. A. Donnelly, N. M. Ferguson, M. E. J. Woolhouse, C. J. Watt, H. J. Udy, S. MaWhinney, et al. 1996. Transmission dynamics and epidemiology of BSE in British cattle. *Nature* **382**, 779–88.

Cousens, S. N., E. Vynnycky, M. Zeidler, R. G. Will, P. G. Smith 1997. Predicting the CJD epidemic in humans. *Nature* **385**, 197–8.

Curnow, R. N., W. V. S. Wijeratne, C. M. Hau 1993. The inheritance of susceptibility to BSE. Proceedings of EC Consultation on transmissible spongiform encephalopathies. Brussels 109–24.

Dealler, S. F. 1993. Bovine spongiform encephalopathy (BSE): The potential effect of the epidemic on the human population. *British Food Journal* **95**(8), 22–34.

Dealler, S. F. 1996. *House of Commons Select Committee on Agriculture and Health, April 1996.* London: HMSO.

Dealler, S. F., J. T. Kent 1995. BSE: an update on the statistical evidence. *British Food Journal* **97**(8), 3–18.

Editorial 1996. The hazards of Government data. *Nature* **383**, 463.

Foster, J. D., M. Bruce, L. McConnell, A. Chree, H. Fraser 1996. Detection of BSE infectivity in brain and spleen of experimentally infected sheep. *Veterinary Record* **138**, 546–8.

Marsh, R. F. 1990. Bovine spongiform encephalopathy in the United States. *Journal of the American Veterinary Medicine Association* **196**, 1677–8.

Ministry of Agriculture Fisheries and Food 1996a. *Bovine spongiform encephalopathy in Great Britain. A progress report, May 1996.* London: MAFF.

Ministry of Agriculture Fisheries and Food 1996b. *Programme to eradicate BSE in the United Kingdom. May 1996.* London: MAFF.

Owen, J. B. 1996. Bovine spongiform encephalopathy (BSE) – a review of causes and state of present knowledge. In *BSE. The Welsh Dimension*. J. Bristow (ed.), 11–22. Cardiff: Institute of Welsh Affairs and the Welsh Institute of Rural Studies.

Spongiform Encephalopathy Advisory Committee 1996. *Statement on maternal transmission of BSE. August 1996*. London: MAFF.

Appendix 1

BSE cases reported outside Great Britain (May 1996)

Northern Ireland	1705
Isle of Man	464
Jersey	120
Guernsey	564
Alderney	2
Republic of Ireland	124
France	20
Portugal	37
Switzerland	214
Germany	4
Denmark	1
Italy	2
Canada	1
Oman	1
Falkland Islands	1

Appendix 2

Number of confirmed cases of BSE: within-herd incidences and numbers of new herds with BSE (results from MAFF, UK)

	Within herd incidence		No. of new herds
	Jan–Jun	Jul–Dec	with BSE
1986–88	1.8	1.8	2582
1989	2.0	1.9	3824
1990	2.1	2.2	4802
1991	2.3	2.5	5970
1992	2.7	2.7	7264
1993	2.5	2.4	5457
1994	2.3	2.3	2383
1995	2.1	1.9	1107

Chapter 5

Chronic Uncertainty and BSE Communications: Lessons from (and Limits of) Decision Theory

Paul Anand

Introduction

In terms of public debate, mad cow disease (bovine spongiform encephalopathy or BSE) comes close to being the AIDS crisis the UK never had. Described by John Major as the most testing problem of his time as prime minister, BSE is an important potential health risk, but is even more significant as a *symbolic public occasion* which society uses to work through how it wants *such issues handled*. Although openness and litigiousness are not defining characteristics of the UK context (both are on the rise), there are several quite general lessons that emerge from the country's experience since BSE became an issue of public concern in 1986.

From a decision–theoretic perspective, one of the major problems that BSE highlights is the difficulty of decision making and risk regulation under conditions of radical uncertainty. Indeed some commentators emphasize the fact that we still have little idea about the future consequences for public health in the UK (in particular what will happen to statistics for deaths from Creutzfeldt–Jakob disease (CJD)). However, it is worth recognizing that after various epidemiological investigations and research exercises we now do know more than we did at the onset of BSE. By contrast, the early months (if not years) of this "crisis" were characterized by profound ignorance of causes, consequences or remedies, yet it is under such conditions that the all-important early decisions had to be made. Indeed uncertainty is almost a defining characteristic of the beginning of any public health scare – the major variation being in how long the uncertainty lasts.

As a complement to many of the commentaries that deal with relatively recent events, I want, in this chapter, to examine the extent to which a decision–theoretic perspective can help understand the problems of decision making without the information or evidence that one would, ideally, want. In doing this, the chapter draws on a comparative analysis[1] of the government's management of the BSE food crisis (see Anand & Forshner 1995), to highlight some decision making and information related issues of general relevance to those involved in the communication[2] of food- and health-related issues. In addition, we shall also identify some limits to the applicability of decision theory in the food health scares which BSE illustrates so well.

The chapter takes the following structure. Section 2 introduces two theoretical issues: the first is a distinction between risk (where probabilities are known) and uncertainty (where probabilities are unknown), and the second is a set of decision-making frameworks that might provide a normative basis for decision making in health risk or food scare contexts. Section 3 provides a brief description of BSE (as a case study) within a multi-stage model of the public construction of food scares. Section 4 goes on to discuss BSE in terms of different decision-making approaches actually used and concludes with some lessons for future practice.

What can Economic Decision Theory Contribute?

Experience seems to suggest that the distinction between risk and uncertainty (found in decision theory) is critical to understanding the early stages of many health risk problems. Often attributed to the research of the economist Frank Knight (1921) and more recently related to work in Keynes' (1921) *A Treatise on Probability*,[3] the distinction is illustrated in the decision problem in Table 5.1.

In the decision problem described in Table 5.1, the gold-standard approach to decision making under risk – expected utility – selects the option that yields the highest probability weighed sum of utilities. One could measure utility in terms of expected life-years (say), but people may prefer small sure gains to large expected gains with a substantial downside risk, and typically they differ in their sensitivity to such risks. Expected utility is capable of capturing these differential sensitivities to risk, and a variety of patterns are well known: we can easily describe people who are risk averse, risk preferring, or some combination of the two. Evidence suggests, for example, that many people are risk averse when the outcomes are positive, but that they are risk preferring when the outcomes are losses. For repeated decisions, there is less need to be sensitive to risk – the gains and losses tend to cancel out, and this is a perspective often relevant to those who take risks on a regular basis.

Table 5.1 Payoffs for acts under different unknown states

	High human risk	Medium human risk	Humans immune
Ban UK beef	0.9	0.5	0.1
Target infective material	0.4	0.6	0.2
Status quo	0.0	0.1	1.0

The entries in the act–state matrix above represent positive utilities. A wide variety of patterns are possible depending on underlying assumptions about what is and is not valuable. Here the utilities are scaled from 0 (worst) to 1 (best).

However, there are many decisions that do not, to the bearer of risk, appear to be replicable. Cohen (1995), for example, recently argued that expected utility might not apply to medical decisions because, although treatment decisions are repeated across patients by medical experts, patients frame their own treatment decision as a one-shot problem. Even in one-shot problems, a decision maker might sometimes have probabilistic information though some such problems might be sufficiently novel that there are either too few or two many probability distributions that plausibly could be relevant and in these cases a different formal structure for decision making under uncertainty is more appropriate.

The practical value of the literature on decision making under uncertainty[4] is to be found in the different rules it identifies. One can select that option that has the best, worst payoff (maximin) or more optimistically, the option which has the best, highest payoff (maximax). In the example in Table 5.1, "targeting infective material" – the action taken by the UK government in 1989 – is the maximin choice. One can use a combination of the two rules (the Hurwicz criterion) or it can be assumed that all states are equally likely, and calculate an expected utility accordingly. All these approaches are the subject of normative debate (Luce & Raiffa 1957), but it is important to note that no one rule has emerged as more acceptable than any others. In decision making under uncertainty therefore (e.g. in the early stage of some health crisis where causal mechanisms are poorly understood) there is considerable scope for parties to disagree about what should be done. In a sense, this is a negative finding – people look to decision theory to say how they should choose and here decision theory seems to be saying that you can rationalize any choice depending on your level of optimism or pessimism. What this shows is that even disinterested decision makers might, quite legitimately, take very different views about what to do.

A second set of issues that merit consideration relate to different possible ways of framing a decision. There are several mathematical frameworks that provide a basis for decision making under uncertainty and these are summarized in Table 5.2.

I describe each of these frameworks in more detail elsewhere,[5] though most will be familiar. Normally decision theorists work within one of the frameworks above and seek to determine within an experimental set-up what kind of decision rules people use.

The question we ask here, however, is what kind of framework is being used in public debate to analyse the decision problems associated with BSE (the main one being whether to allow continued human consumption of UK beef).

Table 5.2 Possible normative frameworks for uncertain health problems

Uncertainty/Ambiguity	Multi-attribute Utility
Decision Trees	Benefit–Cost Analysis
Quantitative Risk Analysis	Social Choice (e.g. voting or polling)
Bayesian Updating	Negotiation

This larger set of frameworks allows us to cater for the possibility that key players might be using a decision-making framework which is neither risk nor uncertainty based. Prior to doing the research we saw this as a set of potentially competing hypotheses relating to problem framing though, as we shall see, they appear to be more complementary than the standard accounts suggest.

Although we conducted some quantitative analysis of the public debate, many of the more important issues emerge more clearly from an interpretative analysis of events, and for that reason the next section centers around a qualitative discussion of several issues.

The Case of BSE

This section presents some details of the case within a stage model of a food crisis. Some of the stages might be expected to follow sequentially, others will vary depending on the case (especially components of stage 3). Each stage, however, marks a new episode in which the demands being made of decision makers and communicators can be expected to change. These stages can be found in the salmonella-in-eggs scare of the late 1980s (see Forshner 1993), although based on these two comparative studies it seems that the importance of the different stages (as well as the sequence) is likely to vary depending on the particular issue. Clearly what we present provides only one example and a conceptualization which needs to be tested on a larger sample before statistical generalizations can be made. That said, I believe practitioners involved in such episodes will readily identify with many of the stages as ones they have had to work through themselves.

Stage 1. Quirky science

Early coverage[6] of BSE in 1986–7 was slim, and what discussion there was concerned the relation between BSE in cattle and scrapie in sheep. Scrapie is a nervous disorder that has been endemic in the UK sheep flock for some 250 years with no apparent effect on humans. Although this may not be true for deliberations within government, early media coverage focused almost exclusively on understanding the natural science. There is little if any discussion of the effects on industry or consumers, or the possible financial consequences for taxpayers. At that time, and for reasons that reflect the interests of political journalists in the UK, BSE was basically a "science story".

Stage 2. "Do something"

Although the government had introduced various policies in 1988,[7] public interest (proxied by media coverage) first became substantial immediately prior to publication of the Southwood Report. It contained various recommendations for action which the government announced that it would implement in full, although it took some months to do so.

One of the more common criticisms is that the government was not reacting quickly enough – criticisms which can pressure politicians into setting up committees, inquiries and so on that may generate more reports than action, but which nonetheless create an opportunity within government where resources are freed up slightly and refocused on the task at hand. Indeed, it is striking just how frequently criticisms concerning speed of response are made: perhaps they are easy to make.

Stage 3a. Stakeholder spread

To examine the nature of stakeholder involvement, we examined the different kinds of stakeholders whose views were reported. Figure 5.1 compares the number of stakeholder categories[8] with (a proxy for) the level of coverage. Clearly one would expect a greater range of stakeholders to be involved as coverage increases, but in this case it appears that once different stakeholder categories are drawn into the debate, they stay there.

Stage 3b. Playing off the experts

The *bête noire* of the BSE story is (or was) a professor of microbiology at Leeds University. Early on in the debate he took a position that put him in conflict with government when he emphasized a very worst-case scenario in which millions of people might die. The government's response was not enthusiastic, but the more dismissive the government's reaction the better established, it

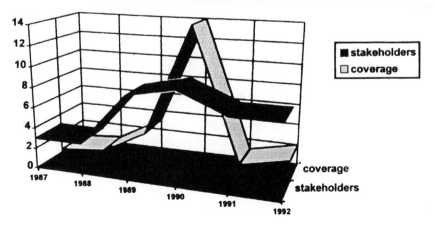

Figure 5.1 Stakeholder references and coverage.

seemed, the professor became as the focal expert the media would play off against government pronouncements. However, by 1996, there seemed to be some recognition in the press that there was no-one who really knew whether, for example, humans could contract CJD from eating contaminated meat or, if so, how infectious contaminated material might be. This acknowledgment of what might be regarded as radical uncertainty undercuts the game of playing off experts, as there are no facts and therefore nothing (as the media see it) for anyone to be an expert about.

Stage 3c. Internationalization

In 1990, US servicemen based in the UK were banned from eating beefburgers made with UK produced beef. The direct financial losses to the industry were, in and of themselves, trivial though the symbolic value was potentially much greater. Government politicians did try to suggest the move was a form of "retaliation" for UK bans of hormone-treated beef – a ban that had seemed equally ill-founded to American beef producers. A couple of years later, Moscovites were concerned about food aid from the UK in case the meat had come from BSE contaminated beef – and they had to be reassured that this was not the case by the Minister for Overseas Affairs. However, many countries around the world outside the European Community (EC) and not subject to EC law banned the import of UK beef, and there was very little the government seemed able to do about this. These actions serve as a motion of no confidence in a government though they did not, as it happens, have much impact on the British public's evaluation of the safety of UK beef or, for that matter, the adequacy of the government's response.

Stage 3d. Regulatory conflict

This seems to occur both within a country and between countries. We have already touched on international aspects – for countries who have their own producers, it is particularly popular to ban imports where there is the slightest suggestion of a food risk problem. In the UK, local food quality among other things comes under the purview of local trading standards officers, although on at least one occasion we have found evidence of a member of parliament making a statement (concerning the entry of contaminated animals entering the human food chain) contradicting evidence produced by trading standards officers only one week before. Within Europe, the European Commission has played a major role more recently[9] when it tried to bring a negotiated settlement between countries (like the UK and Germany) that have different beliefs about safety, public confidence, and remedial action. However the Commission is not a court of law and the UK government's policy of non-cooperation in EC business at ministerial level in the middle of 1996 illustrates some of the problems of international risk regulation in a context where there is no natural equivalent to a final court of appeal.

Stage 4. Issue redefinition

Researchers have identified a process of "social amplification" as crises develop over time, and BSE (as a social issue) has certainly become discussed well beyond the bounds of agriculture. BSE has also become a different issue, and during 1996, following the reported increase in CJD statistics associated with younger victims, emphasis has shifted from *beef industry concerns* to those of *public health*. The rise in CJD statistics (statistical significance apart) provides a factual basis on which the issue is elevated in importance and the fact that government health ministers now speak on the issue reflects this definitional change in what Price (1996) calls the "rational structure" of the problem. Issue redefinition is of particular significance as it brings with it a new set of priorities and implicit understandings about the appropriate mechanisms by which decisions should be made.

In a sense, this goes to the heart of how we handle and discuss potential healthcare crises. What kind of issue we believe something is, defines what kind of expertise we accept as relevant. The public-health perspective was relatively underrepresented in BSE communications until recently, although the actions taken *do* suggest the government was certainly concerned about public-health issues. One can speculate that the government might have won more credit for its actions had it chosen to frame them as defending public health, rather than supporting or "being fair" to farmers.

Stage 5. "Do more"

Initially officials pointed to 1992 being a crucial year for BSE statistics. In fact the numbers of cattle infected declined, as did media interest, until the statistics for human CJD victims began to take over. The EC again became involved, and pressure mounted on the UK government to take steps which most people regarded as being of symbolic value (culling animals over 30 months in age). In mid-1996, the results of research into maternal transmission of BSE instigated in 1989 showed that this was indeed a possibility and helped to heighten pressure for further action. When the experiment was commissioned (in 1989) it rather looked as if its results might emerge years after the whole affair had gone away, and yet it shows how early attempts to "do the right thing" and allay public concerns can have secondary counterproductive effects several years on.

Stage 6. Process redefinition

Following the salmonella-in-eggs crisis, a parliamentary select committee (comprising backbenchers from a range of parties) criticized the Ministry for Agriculture, Fisheries and Food (MAFF) for the extent to which it had listened to industry concerns about their own costs and profits. In its 1990 report on BSE, however, the committee noted that MAFF had taken an apparently more "scientific" approach and congratulated them for doing so. Major crises have an impact on the way similar problems are handled in the future, although without a theoretical framework one is left with intuitively plausible reactions that may well be counterproductive. From a decision–theoretic viewpoint the ideal is to integrate information on consequences and likelihoods, whereas the government response seems to have shifted from one incomplete information source to another.

Analysis and Lessons

In terms of our initial hypothesis about decision making under uncertainty, the story reviewed supports the view that an uncertainty framework is relevant. Certainly most of the early communications did not reflect a low subjective probability of risk but rather a categorical judgment of acceptability – UK beef is safe. In some cases, for example in discussions over power safety, experts have been willing to say that risks were one in a million, although however "authoritative" the expert is, this is still an expression of a subjective probability (it cannot be a relative frequency, for example).

Possibly stronger evidence for an uncertainty interpretation is the weight given to the absence of causal knowledge about transmission mechanisms and verified demonstrations of transmission to humans. These lacunae were taken to be reason to discount the risk to humans, although we should be careful about the meaning of phrases like "no scientific evidence" which are used often in contexts such as this. If what is meant is that rigorous scientific work shows there is no statistical risk, then perhaps we might be reassured. If, on the other hand, this means all the evidence so far is only anecdotal, or that it is too early to expect to attribute statistical significance to the differences that we are observing, or even that no scientist has looked at this problem yet, then reassurance is surely inappropriate.

Inappropriateness of Hypothesis Testing

(a) Sparse data

We find no evidence in the public debate that the *process* of decision making is the subject of consultation with appropriate experts.[10] Instead, advice on appropriate decision-making techniques comes predominately on the back of natural science advice and is therefore normally related to the framework for the statistical testing of hypotheses. Hypothesis testing, however, is notoriously inappropriate for situations where data is sparse, yet this is just the situation that needs to be handled.

(b) Absence of belief–payoff integration

A second reason why hypothesis testing is inappropriate (as usually practiced) is that it makes no explicit allowance for payoffs. In the normal course of events, the decision to reject or accept an observed difference is dependent on purely epistemic criteria, the sample size, the sampling distribution under the null hypothesis and the alternative hypothesis. There is no room for what's at stake, and while this may be appropriate for theory testing, it cannot be helpful in contexts where the consequences of type 1 and type 2 errors vary dramatically.

For both reasons the use of hypothesis testing as a framework for decision making under uncertainty is undesirable. Decision making under uncertainty is the closest formal framework (scenario planning the management counterpart). However, as we noted, a defining feature of ambiguity in practice is the absence of knowledge and demonstrative proof, neither of which feature in the conceptual framework of decision theory. The omission is a serious weakness for decision theory.

Actions Worth Considering

1. Understand media and institutional filters

Much attention has gone into understanding public perceptions, but the public debate is driven by the media's reaction to its anticipation and perceptions of public interest, not public perceptions directly. While one might sympathize with policy-makers' difficulties in handling the press, it seems that only recognition of the media as a legitimate and distinct stakeholder (rather than as a mere informational conduit) will lead to a proper understanding of its behavior which is predictable, though not necessarily correlated with any objective assessment of risk.

2. Survey public concerns

Notwithstanding the above, it seems useful to take steps to maintain some *ongoing* understanding of public concerns, independent of their reflection in the tinted windows of media coverage. The factors underlying perception include size of hazard, ambiguity, and perceived voluntariness of risk-bearing, but these are not sufficient to understand why the public want some risks to be regulated more than others. Questions of trust in organizations also seem to play an important role (Pidgeon et al. 1993).

3. Develop fast-track information systems

During the early years of the BSE problem, information about research seemed to emerge in a rather haphazard way and often after the enquiries of journalists.

On-line records of research have improved considerably since the late 1980s and these should make it much easier to locate relevant research, years after its completion, even when funded by different government bodies.

4. Establish a risk communication strategy

Recently in the UK, the Health and Safety Executive (1996) have published the deliberations of a working group looking at risk assessment across government departments. They acknowledged the need to address risk communication issues in the UK and concluded that a more open, consistent approach was needed and that, given time, members of the public do make sensible judgments based on scientific evidence. However, without some model of the communication process and its aims and objectives, it is hard to say whether greater emphasis on risk communication will lead to improved communicative efforts.

Calls for more openness are hard to disagree with (at least in the UK context), but it is questionable whether interdepartmental consistency should be the number one priority. If one takes the view, for instance, that trust in organizations is critical to the success of attempts to provide reassurance, then perhaps the most important feature of a communication strategy is how one deals with the establishment of good working relations with key institutional filters (like the media) on a day-to-day basis. Given also the dependence of risk acceptability on a variety of factors, it seems that perhaps the most important is the requirement to develop risk communication policies appropriate to particular kinds of risks as the public see them.

5. Re-evaluate the role of politicians

Although political involvement in the UK government is limited to decisions made at the highest levels, it is still not clear that the contribution is positive and/or necessary. The prime-time TV pictures of John Gummer[11] feeding his four-year-old daughter a beefburger brought only criticism. Given that the politicians usually bring no particular science or social science expertise to their role (except perhaps from law or business), it is questionable whether they are in a position to judge what kind of expertise is appropriate. Nevertheless they do make final decisions in high profile cases, and in some instances these decisions amount to much more (or less) than the mere rubber stamping of work done by ministry officials. It is easy to see how expertise becomes valuable in a system characterized by countervailing powers, less so in a hierarchical one presided over by generalists.

In mid-1996, a major tobacco producer took out a paid advertisement in the *Guardian* (a UK "quality" daily newspaper) pointing out that the risks from second-hand smoke were about the same as those from eating one biscuit a day. In general, the government has avoided making such facile comparisons and its actions may, in years to come, be regarded as appropriate. There seems to be a consensus, however, that communicative efforts have not been so successful. *If that judgement is fair, then I would argue that it is due, not to individual incompetence, but rather to an inappropriate Whitehall–Westminster culture that places more faith in natural science working behind closed doors than is currently appropriate given the expectations about the transparency of policy and the responsiveness of policy-makers.*

Notes

1 We have compared BSE with the outbreak of salmonella-in-eggs, but concentrated here on the former issue.
2 Following the inadequacy of one-way and even two-way communication models, it is common to define communication broadly enough so that it includes political and other forms of social negotiation.
3 The most thorough discussion of Keynes' views on the distinction between uncertainty and risk appears in Runde (1990).
4 A theoretical review appears in Kelsey (1988).
5 The framework is discussed also by (the late) Barry Turner (1994).
6 Our data refers to coverage in *The Times* of London. It is (or was) the paper of record and as BSE became politicized along party lines only recently, coverage has up to now been rather similar in the UK qualities. Other work we are doing on newspaper coverage of healthcare reforms suggests that the political colour of a newspaper is reflected in the sometime quite subtle slants put on stories. Otherwise, we find that *The Times* and the *Guardian* (the spreadsheet paper aligned to the left) very often cover the same stories.
7 Ruminant feed ban (18 July), slaughter policy (8 August), destruction of milk legislation (30 December): Source, Agriculture Committee (1990).
8 The categories of stakeholders identified are: government representatives, government scientists, medical or industry experts, retailers, public or consumer groups, farmer representatives, beef dealers and producers, EC officials, and representatives of other governments.
9 This comment was written in mid-1996.
10 If one allows the employment of advertising agencies then there is evidence of professional advice being sought in the communication sphere.
11 His brother is a public relations expert in the UK.

References

Anand, P. & C. Forshner 1995. Of mad cows and marmosets. *British Journal of Management* **6**, 221–33.
Agriculture Committee 1990. *Bovine spongiform encephalopathy*. Fifth Report 1989–1990. London: HMSO.

Cohen, B. J. 1996. Is expected utility theory normative for medical decision-making? *Medical Decision Making* **16**, 1–6.

Forshner, C. 1993. *The British government, mad cows and rotten eggs.* MPhil thesis, University of Oxford.

Health and Safety Executive 1996. *Use of risk assessment within government departments.* London: HSE.

Kelsey, D. 1988. *A survey of ignorance.* Discusson paper, Churchill College Cambridge.

Keynes, J. M. 1921. *A treatise on probability.* London: Macmillan.

Knight, F. 1921. *Risk uncertainty and profit.* Boston: Houghton Mifflin.

Luce, D. & H. Raiffa 1957. *Games and decisions.* New York: John Wiley.

Pidgeon, N. et al. 1993. Risk perception. In *Risk.* London. Royal Society.

Price, D. 1996. Lessons for health care rationing from the case of Child B. *British Medical Journal* **312**, 167–9.

Runde, J. 1990. Keynesian uncertainty and the weight of arguments. *Economics and Philosophy* **6**, 275–92.

Turner, B. 1994. The future of risk research. *Journal of Contingencies and Crisis Management* **2**, 146–56.

Part II

Politics as Health

Chapter 6

BSE and CJD: Recent Developments

Tim Lang

Introduction

The following paper was prepared as written evidence to the House of Commons joint Agriculture and Health Committees' hearings into BSE (bovine spongiform encephalopathy) (Agriculture and Health Committees 1997) to which I also gave verbal witness. The Committees' unprecedented joint hearings were a disappointment. Both verbal and written evidence were published but no report from the committees was generated. This silence was regrettable and a set-back for those who argued that the Select Committee could be a useful democratic brake on Government. If nothing else, a crisis as significant as BSE surely warranted a considered set of recommendations from the all-party committees.

Although regrettable, perhaps the silence was understandable. The questions raised by BSE go to the heart of contemporary food production. Was this epidemic merely a failure of management, the lessons of which can be incorporated into a continued system of intensive production, or was it their death knell? Was the loss of public confidence in Government a peculiar difficulty of the MAFF's (Ministry of Agriculture, Fisheries and Food) close relations with producers, or was this the kind of nightmare that could face any government supposedly responsible for public safety in a highly complex economic sector? These are complex questions, requiring a more open mind than the Committees were apparently prepared, or allowed, to make.

Since I wrote the paper, the questions and crisis have intensified rather than diminished. The European Parliament has produced a highly criticized report – of both the British Government and the European Commission (EC) – which has led to an important speech on 18 February 1997 by Jacque Santer, the EU (European Union) President (Santer 1997). Mr Santer's speech acknowledged that this was a crisis over whether the market was being put before considerations of public health. He promised reforms of how the Commission would operate in the future. Specifically, he promised: a separation of regulation from promotion of industry and of legislation from inspection; more "transparency", that Euro-word for open government!; and the creation of a new food agency under a strengthened Consumer Affairs Directorate, D-G XXIV and separate from the all-powerful Agriculture Directorate D-G VI.

Mr Santer stated that the BSE crisis had important lessons for the direction for reforming the Common Agricultural Policy. "Can we really go on claiming that BSE is an accident of nature?" he asked. "Is it not actually the consequence of a model of agricultural production which pushes productivity at whatever cost?" (Santer 1997: para 12). If followed through, this could be a significant shift in EU agriculture policy, away from agriculture and towards food, something the present author has long argued for (Lang 1992, Lang et al. 1996). Indeed, Mr Santer actually called for "the gradual establishment of a proper food policy which gives pride of place to consumer protection and consumer health."

Would that such thoughts had emanated from the Conservative British Government in the same open manner. In the year since I wrote this memorandum to the Committees, Government policy remained one of damage limitation rather than forward looking. In the wake of continued revelations about meat hygiene, the political process began to move. In particular, the case for reforming the Ministry of Agriculture intensified. The Labour Party and Liberal Democrats both promised to set up a food agency and the Conservatives promised a new Chief Food Safety Officer and a new, non-executive, Food Safety Council. The debate, in other words, was no longer whether to change the organs of Government but how to. In the event Labour won the 1997 election by a landslide. There is to be a new agency up and running by 1999. There will also be a new risk committee at the Department of Health.

Besides these institutional and policy shifts, both in line with what was written here, one other point is significant. The distinction this memorandum made between risk management and a trust relationship has become more widely accepted. Risk assessment with its "top down" managerial assumptions has been shown to be inapplicable in situations such as BSE. Food implies a trust relationship as well as a risk relationship. Research by the Centre for the Study of Environmental Change at Lancaster University on genetically modified organisms in the food chain has confirmed the suggestion made here that consumers are both more wary and more rational in their behavior than the risk assessment model allows (Grove-White et al. 1997).

Consumers are too often put into narrow psychological boxes by food policy discourse when in fact they are more sophisticated and complex (Gabriel & Lang 1995). Meanings attached to food are so wide-ranging that there is plenty of scope for contradictions and subtlety alongside clarity and purpose. This new more complex approach to consumers has enormous implications for producers and retailers. They are being forced to re-think their responsibility for product safety and, having resisted it for years, are rapidly introducing a notion of "traceability". It remains to be seen how extensive this becomes. Pressure for more open information, not just about products but about the processes which occur before the consumer sees them, are likely to intensify. Studies of labeling policy and practice have suggested that despite the rhetoric of consumer sovereignty, information given to consumers about food is severely limited (Black & Rayner 1992, Lang 1995).

The impact of the BSE outbreak and its possible connection to new variant-Creutzfeldt–Jakob disease (v-CJD) has already been immense. It is presently unclear where this will lead food policy. Rather like the process of breaking a log-jam in a river, the BSE crisis has exposed for all eyes to see the power of the competing interests in the hugely profitable but necessary food market. Who knows whether one outcome might even be more influence for consumers? Certainly, the power brokers of the old order, from politicians to producers, now know that all eyes are on them. Those naïve scientists who used to argue that consumers merely needed to be made more literate and that politicians should implement their verdicts also have learned some humility. In uncertain areas of science, it is a fool who professes perfect vision.

Memorandum to the House of Commons Joint Agriculture and Health Committees' hearings into BSE

Summary and Recommendations

BSE has provided an object lesson in how not to manage risk. Eight years into the crisis, too much attention has been paid to too narrow a conception of science and not enough attention has been paid to failings of public policy with regard to consumers, decision making at MAFF and information flow to the public. A chasm was opened up in public confidence by the early 1990s, which subsequent events have only widened. This submission argues that improvements in public confidence in beef will only be generated once longer-term reforms are put in place. Proposals are given to this effect.

Several conclusions can be drawn from the above:

(a) It is wrong to look to science to provide answers to social problems. As critics of science throughout the twentieth century have argued, all science can do is make judgements on base of best evidence. Science reflects, but does not transcend, its social context. Ministerial reliance upon science not only misunderstood the nature of science in general but made unwarranted statements about the certainty of current understanding about BSE in particular.

(b) Unless consumers, or their representatives, are involved in judging risk, their behavior is likely to be unmanageable. Indeed, there are strong grounds for arguing that even in low risk situations, heightened awareness that there is a risk can lead to risk avoidance behavior or, as with cigarette smoking, into elaborate rationalizations of chosen patterns of behavior.

(c) Government has been hoist by its narrow conception of research into consumers. It has not apparently drawn upon work it has itself funded. Representatives of consumer, environmental health and social science should be represented on the Spongiform Encephalopathy Advisory Committee (SEAC), and other relevant committees. BSE shows that a narrow view of science will not provide a sufficiently broad base of advice from which government can act sensibly.

(d) There should be a national debate about the role, and case for reform of, the MAFF.

(e) There should be a review of government's approach to consumer information. Consideration should be given to setting up a Consumer Information Unit, but only if it was based upon a policy of listening to, and incorporating consumer concerns. The tone, as well as the substance, of information should be inclusive rather than patronizing.

(f) No reform process would be complete without a commitment to change direction in national food and farming policy away from further intensification, and towards a more extensive, sustainable system of production. This has been argued for on environmental grounds, now also on public health and consumer confidence grounds.

(g) The immediate task of reducing the incidence of BSE should take note of the Agriculture Committee's advice in its 1990 report, when it argued that government should go beyond what the scientists say "whether for political, commercial or other reasons". As consumers now know, the government ignored that advice too. No resolution is possible without following that earlier advice.

(h) Behind this sorry saga is a wider, moral truth. Food should not be for ever treated as the output of an industrial process. Nature is not to be raided and pillaged. This is a crisis of industrialized food and farming. Diseased bits of dead sheep were fed to herbivores which humans then ate. Labeling should include more information about not just the content of the food, but of the process which generated it.

(i) There should be an independent inquiry into the feedstuff industry, and the rendering industry in particular. Taxpayers' support for the renderers should be conditional upon reform.

1. Introduction: Juggling competing interests

MAFF has had the difficult task of juggling competing interests over BSE. These interests included: defence of the meat industry, public health, consumer confidence, its own reputation, cost, making decisions in a difficult scientific context and, last but not least, government ideology (particularly on supporting industry).

We know that this juggling act has failed. As a result, MAFF has entered the annals of food and public policy history as being the first ministry to help devastate an industry it is in existence to promote. The Select Committees need to decide why this happened. My own judgement is that MAFF and the Government placed an unwarranted reliance upon an evolving scientific understanding of BSE, and that when drastic action such as a culling program in the early days was appropriate, backed off.

Action was not taken, despite a covert recommendation from the Agriculture Committee in 1990, among others, to do so, out of a short-sighted belief that that would be an unnecessarily harsh punishment on the meat industries. Paragraphs 43 and 44 of the 1990 Agriculture Committee report should still be implemented. These argued that the Government should go beyond what the scientists say "whether for political, commercial or other reasons".

As a consequence, certain sections of the food industries have been hammered even harder than they would have been from 1989 on, and the government is now in the embarrassing position of trying to provide financial and other support to a considerable extent – with or without European backing. Annual culling and compensation costs from now on of up to £0.5 billion are no mean bill to pay for a policy mistake.

Government has argued consistently (see section 4 on risk below) that the foundation for its policy is science. This is not the whole picture. Although knowledge about spongiform encephalopathies is by no means new (see, for example, Gajdusek's comprehensive review in 1985, before the UK BSE crisis emerged), it is evolving fast and despite large sums of research money is still not, in the words of one writer in the recent *British Medical Journal* series of articles, "as robust as once thought" (Roberts 1995).

The Government underestimated the significance of three factors in the policy arena which became critical: (1) the role of consumers and information in the marketplace; (2) the contradictions in MAFF's role in food policy; and (3) the nature and perception of risk.

Hard questions need to be asked of each of these, as to whether the Government was given advice. If it was, what was it? If it wasn't, why not?

2. Information and the consumer

BSE was a terrible shock to consumers and farmers alike, but it has had the effect of bringing them closer together. Consumers who had been worried about modern farming practices, on occasions accusing them of adulterating food (London Food Commission 1988) being excessively subsidized (National Consumers Council 1988) and polluting the land, (for example, see Maynard 1991) began to have sympathy for them.

Consumer confidence the key

Polls suggest that support for farmers would be high if farming was to be conducted in more ecologically sustainable and socially acceptable directions. In an NOP poll in February 1992, 71 per cent said there need to be more control in the methods farmers use; 82 per cent said they favoured an increase in organic farming; 79 per cent said taxpayers' support should only go to farmers who farm in ways that do not harm the environment; 83 per cent saying taxpayers' support should only go to farmers who do not harm animal welfare (see Safe Alliance 1992). Farmers, who had at times seen consumers as necessary but ill-informed evils, found themselves to have been fraudulently treated as consumers of the feedstuffs industry. Both parties have been rendered victims by contaminated material being fed to cattle.

BSE has changed the food policy landscape within which consumers think, act, and eat. The disease has entered everyday language, featuring in jokes and references for years. The current situation, therefore, may have come as a surprise to people elsewhere in the world, but not to British consumers. There have been countless TV programmes and newspapers articles on the subject since news first broke.

People, in my experience, are generally sober and sensible about the subject, although the scale of the epidemic is clearly considerable. Approximately 160,000 cows have suffered from the disease which now affects 34.4 per cent of British farms (MAFF 1995:4) – 53.3 per cent of dairy farms, but only 14.7 of beef suckler herds (Gore 1995).

Although from an early stage, Government informed consumers that it knew what the disease's cause was – infected feed – scientists were simultaneously asking many more uncertain questions (see the list of research suggestions in the 1989 Tyrrell Report) (Consultative Committee on Research into Spongiform Encephalopathies 1989: 5–18). From the very beginning of the BSE saga, therefore, some ambivalence was built into the nature of information on the subject – certainty alongside uncertainty. Industrial and government interests have tended to favour certainty, while consumers to a greater extent asked the "what if" questions more overtly. Science, being a process, not a static state of knowledge, has always suggested less certainty than everyone desired (for example, see Dealler 1996).

Low confidence in Government over food

It should also be recognized that, in such crisis situations, Government is no longer the only source of information in the public arena. One academic study of the food scandals of 1988–90 (in which BSE was part) found that non-Government figures were as significant, if not more so, in media appearances, than Government ministers (Miller & Reilly 1994).

Public confidence is a key factor in crises, yet the Government has seriously misjudged and mishandled it, exacerbating consumer volatility and engendering entirely understandable behavior which went against Government's stated intentions.

The BSE crisis emerged at the end of a decade in which the Government has already been severely dented with regard to its handling of food policy: salmonella, listeria, microwave oven safety, food irradiation, additives; the list seemed long. In July 1989, at the height of the food scandals – with BSE only recently in the public arena – the Consumers Association conducted a poll; three out of four people agreed with the statement "the Government has failed to protect consumers from unsafe food" (poll conducted by Research Surveys of Great Britain, July 1989; quoted in Consumers Association 1991:2). Seven years later, a similar ICM poll for the *Guardian* found attitudes hardening, in that 73 per cent of consumers felt that "the Government knew there was a risk and tried to hide it" (see Linton & Bates 1996:1).

Food labeling: process as well as content

In economic theory, market efficiency depends upon there being many consumers offered goods and services by many producers, and upon there being open and sound information between them. In practice, even food labeling has become a battleground of interests, rather than an effective tool for market efficiency (Lang 1995). Food labeling is limited to the list of contents (in decreasing order by weight) and, lately, nutrition information. Even the latter is contentious in that, according to research funded by MAFF (Black & Rayner 1992), it is given in the form least wanted, understood or liked by consumers.

More effort and space is accorded to brand information than process or content labeling; hence the considerable public distaste when it transpired that so many consumer products contain beef products (cosmetics, pharmaceuticals, as well as non-meat foods) (Lobstein 1996). Having been told by MAFF that everything consumers need is on food labels (MAFF), public anger and irritation was understandable when it transpired that it was not.

Over recent years, there has been considerable resistance – led by industry and without apparent strong resistance from MAFF – to giving full disclosure of process information, now being so strongly called for by the public to enable them to avoid products with beef by-products in them. The Food Advisory Committee, for instance, argued strongly against pesticide information in 1991, giving the extraordinary argument that if consumers were worried about pesticide residues, they could always buy organic produce (Food Advisory Committee 1991). Such arguments missed the case for positive declaration – upon which market efficiency relies – and they also ignored the precedent set by the E-numbering system for additive declarations, introduced by the European Commission in the early 1980s.

MAFF also consistently argued against labeling of irradiated foods from 1985, but did, to its credit, bow to pressure in the 1990s when the process was finally legalized. On genetically engineered foods, the Polkinghorne Report did recommend some labeling, but only for transgenic food products where there might be either a health or ethical concern (Polkinghorne 1994). A recent review of surveys of consumer attitudes on biotechnology has shown that consumers want clear and comprehensive labeling about process as well as content (Genetics Forum 1996). Consumers have so far not got this. This should be remedied using new technologies, such as consumer display systems, now available.

The obfuscation and lack of information with regard to BSE is therefore not accidental but happens with regard to other sensitive issues in food. It can be reasonably asserted that this failure is systematic; it happens too regularly for it to be random. It took nearly two decades of medical argument and evidence before even the current inadequate nutrition labeling was introduced. MAFF can with some justice respond that it is not helped by having to negotiate on such matters with other European member states, but the point still stands, that the UK Government reflex is to withhold rather than disclose a wide range of information. MAFF has made some progress, but only when there has been concerted action and campaigning from outside, particularly from non-governmental organizations (NGOs). This culture in MAFF needs to be altered if public confidence is to be won back. Labeling is not the only information failure, however.

Other sources of consumer information

Besides on-food information, the traditional parliamentary model of information flow is something like this: scientists inform ministers and MPs (Members of Parliament); parliamentary debate occurs and the media disseminate it in a kind of "trickle down". This model does not fit well in today's world where the food consumer is barraged with other sources of information. The UK food sector invests in annual sum of approximately £0.6 billion on advertising (Dibb 1993) and is also beginning to move into direct marketing (supermarket "loyalty cards" being but one example of this trend). From the consumer's perspective, politicians' pronouncements on matters relating to food safety are therefore only one among many sources. Although US-style news management – tight, exclusive and task-focused – might work for political news, it is highly inappropriate in consumer affairs.

When consumer confidence is at issue, actions speak louder than words. When Perrier had a problem in February 1990 with benzene contamination at its bottling plant, it withdrew its product worldwide, announced what it was doing and, although it never regained its market position (and was taken over by Nestlé), minimised the damage, and cleaned up the source of contamination (a failure of filtration at the plant to remove the naturally occurring benzene) (BBC Radio 4, "Shelf Lives", 7 May 1996). There was no obfuscation about there being "no risk" coupled with more cautious messages that "more research is needed". The emphasis was upon action to meet consumers' concerns. "No risk" meant removal of the product and cleaning up the source – a classic public health strategy, and not what happened with BSE. There the source remained in flow, but there was an attempt to reassure consumers by assuring them the contamination bits were chanelled away. Whatever its merits or failings scientifically, this was poor consumer psychology.

The Consumer Panel and meeting of chairs of consumer organizations

Learning from other food scandals in 1988–90, MAFF set up its Consumer Panel as another forum for communication. Its value must now be called into doubt. The Panel has often prognosticated on BSE, and free from complicated scientific jargon though these deliberations have been, they have merely been reprises of existing positions; no new light has been cast. The point of relevance now is that the Panel has been completely marginal in Government handling of consumers in this BSE crisis. One could be forgiven for arguing that it is a sop when the heat is off MAFF, and irrelevant when it is.

Although members of the Panel and the quarterly meeting of the minister with chairs of consumer groups were asked to a meeting early on in the crisis, neither body was at the heart of government decision-making or thinking in the immediate aftermath of the BSE crisis. It was not until 14 days after the storm blew that there was a full meeting of the widest number of consumer NGOs with a junior minister, on the invitation of MAFF's head of Consumer Division. What is the point of such information mechanisms if they are "bolt on extras" rather than at the heart of information flow?

Underestimation of consumer power

The Government approached BSE consistently from a narrow perspective, but its fatal mistake was to underestimate consumer knowledge and power. This was ironic, as the Major Government has been particularly forceful in extolling the virtues of consumer sovereignty. It has not a leg to stand on when consumers take them at their word and withdraw their favors from the market place.

For some good to come out of this crisis, there has to be a genuine rather than a cosmetic change in Government thinking with regard to consumers.

The consumer movement has also begun to learn the lessons. Food products, like all objects of consumption, can be highly charged emotionally. Therefore, when a crisis occurs it is never surprising if consumers perceive themselves as victims (Gabriel & Lang 1995). The consumer movement has always been particularly active and popular at times of change in industrial production (Tiemstra 1992).

Trust is a fragile beast. The BSE incident has accelerated scepticism about the food industry. Beef sales were gently declining before the current period and have plummeted since (Irish Food Board survey, quoted in Southey 1996). Before the BSE crisis, the price of beef was only maintained by the rising export of British beef; exports compensating for a declining home market. The hectoring tone adopted by Government on occasions has been counter-productive.

3. MAFF's role in food policy: sponsorship versus regulation

Other factors which the Government has failed to appreciate are the structure of MAFF and the state of food policy in Britain.

The goal of "efficient" farming

The BSE crisis has exposed a conflict in MAFF between its role in promoting an industry and regulating it. Ever since Tom Williams' Agriculture Act 1947, the imperative within MAFF has been to promote "efficient" farming. The lessons of the First and Second World Wars had been learned: firstly, the policy of reliance upon an empire or colonies to provide cheap food was now risky; and secondly, Government has a duty to ensure safe and secure food supplies for all its population (Beveridge 1928, Le Gros Clark & Titmuss 1939, Hammond 1951, Tracy 1982). The 1947 Act symbolized a change of policy and ushered in half a century of application of industrial practices to food and farming. Labor was shed from the land, replaced by the "liquid hoe" and sophisticated machinery; efficiency was judged in financial and gross output terms (Clunes-Ross & Hildyard 1992).

By conventional terms, this revolution on and off the land has been very successful. Yet, 20 years ago, doubts about the efficacy of this industrialization policy began to emerge. The financial, human, and ecological costs began to mount up: loss of biodiversity (Jenkins 1992), pollution of water supplies (Lees & McVeigh 1988), rise of cardiovascular diseases and food-related cancers (World Health Organization 1990), unnecessarily high use of motorways and transport (Raven & Lang 1995), unequal effects on consumers (Leather 1992, Department of Health 1996). Despite growing evidence of public concern, MAFF's policies have continued with only minor adjustment. Conflicts over the definition of "the public interest" emerged into the public arena with increasing regularity and ferocity in the 1980s, beginning with the ill-concealed row in 1982 over the report from the National Advisory Committee on Nutrition Education (NACNE) (Walker & Cannon 1984).

A public perception of MAFF's role grew that, far from being an impartial agent of the national interest, it was to articulate a thinly disguised but deeply ingrained reflex to defend the interests of industry – farmers and food manufacturers (Mills 1992). It would be unfair to accuse one political party of holding a prerogative over this policy; it was shared, albeit more enthusiastically by one than the other (Cannon 1987). The vision of food progress through industrialized efficiency has been common to all Governments since the 1947 Act. It is this vision that has now become the subject of considerable public scepticism, and which lies at the heart of the public reaction to BSE and distrust of Government discussed in the previous section. This distrust is now itself a factor in undermining the capacity of Government to manage the crisis. The public can see, if politicians have not, that narrow definitions of market efficiency led to the recycling of dead, diseased animals and their feeding to herbivores. This was cost-cutting at its most ridiculous.

Reform of MAFF

A review of food and farming policy is long overdue, as is a review of its delivery mechanisms. Lang et al. (1996) argue this case and specifically review some of the key mechanisms of Government food policy. Several options are made for reforming MAFF:

(a) close it down and divide its responsibilities among other ministries (notably the Departments of Health, Trade and Industry, and Environment);

(b) transfer responsibility for food quality and consumer protection to another body (such as the Department of Health or a Food Standards Agency, based on the US, Swedish, or Australian models), leaving the Ministry with an industry promotion remit;

(c) transfer responsibility for agri-industrial promotion to the Department of Trade and Industry, and create a new Ministry of Food;

(d) retain MAFF but radically reform it;

(e) leave it as it is.

The final option, in our view, is undesirable. National debate about these options is overdue and should be conducted on the basis of stated policy objectives. Reform of the Ministry's structure could easily be cosmetic – as happened with the creation of the Food Safety Directorate within MAFF. Initially welcome though that was, recent events have shown that unless wider policy as well as the Ministry's internal culture is changed, consumer confidence will be hard to re-build.

Public confidence will not quickly recover without such action. There are already worrying signs of the BSE crisis being subsumed into a wider, more ideological discourse concerning Britain's place in Europe. While that is understandable, it will do little to resolve the difficulty of regaining public confidence in a food product, public policy and Government. Euroscepticism may or may not be in order, but it will not make people purchase or consume beef.

Intensification and exports: open and closed farming systems
British exports have been seriously affected, and Government policy's reliance on trade liberalisation have been brought up short. There are already serious doubts about the Food from Britain philosophy or exporting more, to compensate for rising food imports. This has measurably harmful environmental effects and doubtful health or economic value (Paxton 1994). This ideological package will lead to ever bigger farms, more intensification and a fragmented rural culture dominated by agribusiness with its eye on world markets rather than on feeding people with a health-enhancing diet (Lang 1966).

The lessons of BSE for food policy point in a different direction. We need more closed systems of farming – farms which produce food from start to finish, which grow their own feedstuffs if possible, which produce food for local markets, and do not just buy in inputs, process them a little, and sell them on. That direction for food production has led us to the absurd situation where cows need a "passport" to ensure consumer confidence. Such certification is desirable to boost short term confidence, but is open to fraud unless tightly monitored. In general, we need shorter, not longer trading routes to build up trust between primary producer and end consumer. Hypermarket power is driving the food economy in precisely the opposite direction (Raven & Lang 1995).

Consumers are also calling for less intensive exploitation of farm animals

(NOP poll for Safe Alliance (1992:4)). More research needs to be done to establish the types of farms BSE appeared on, and their feeding and stocking regimes. BSE has never appeared, for example, on any organic farms, except for two cases where the calves were brought in. Yet MAFF has been extremely reluctant to entertain any policy conclusions.

BSE brings into question the main liberalizing thrust of food policy in Europe for the last 20 years. Just when barriers to trade are coming down across Europe following the Single European Act 1987, and when humans no longer need passports to get between member states, cows now actually have to have one. BSE underlines the necessity for barriers, controls, and restriction of movement. This is not old-fashioned protectionism, but appropriate protection of public health and the policy principle of a government ensuring security of food supply; BSE has undermined that.

The feedstuff industry: why compensate the renderers?

It should also be noted that the feedstuffs industry, in general, and the rendering industry, in particular, got off lightly and deserve rigorous scrutiny. If any other industry has wittingly or unwittingly helped devastate an industry, it would be allowed to go bust. In 1993, the Monopolies and Mergers Commission (MMC) had been critical of the largest renderers for being monopolies. Indeed, involvement by the MMC and the Office of Fair Trading can be traced back further, to the time BSE is supposed to have begun.

In 1985, following an enquiry begun in 1982, the MMC judged that one company, Prosper de Mulder had a monopoly (defined as 25 per cent of a market in UK law), with 44 per cent of market share, yet six years later, the same company's market share had risen to 60 per cent and it was investigated for wanting to take over another company with a 5 per cent market share (Monopolies and Merger Commission 1991). In 1993, the MMC found that Prosper de Mulder had "failed to fulfil certain of the undertakings it gave to the DGFT (Director General of Fair Trading) in 1986 following the MMC's earlier animal waste report" (Department of Trade and Industry 1993). Neil Hamilton, MP, Corporate Affairs Minister, asked the DGFT to seek undertakings that Prosper de Mulder would publish a sample of prices and charges on a weekly basis. In 1995, the MMC further censured the company for "discriminatory pricing".

With this track record, on what moral grounds have the renderers been given a taxpayers' handout of £110 million?

4. Science and the perception of risk

Re-building a public interest ethos

The Government's index of consumer confidence in beef is, it seems, to be measured by beef sales, rather than consumer attitudes, values, or concerns. Attitudes and values could be dismissed as long as the behavior was correct and the cash tills kept ringing. This was a mistake and it is also an unnecessarily crude model of how people thing about, purchase and consume food (Lupton 1996). Food businesses have long learned that consumer confidence has to be earned, not anticipated (AGB Market Intelligence 1989). Government now has to re-learn that same lesson.

Ironically, the British Government's food policy used to be one of the most sophisticated, worldwide, in this respect, mainly due to its experience of relating with, and managing, consumers through the Ministry of Food in the Second World War (Hammond 1951, 1956, 1962; Fenelon 1952). That Ministry was closed and merged into MAFF in the mid-1950s, and much of its public orientation and public health perspective was lost; it is time to recreate that ethos. One mechanism for re-building this within MAFF could be the Minim system (the internal system of objectives) instituted by the present Government. The annual setting of Minim goals should be publicly debated.

The dangers of excessive reliance upon risk assessment: risk vs trust
BSE has highlighted the centrality of risk in public and individual decision making. Risk assessment tools such as HACCP are widely used – for example, in control of food poisoning risks – and have been widely promoted in the UK, following the Food Safety Act 1990. Excessive reliance on the technique can, however, pose risks of a different sort. Companies and Government can easily turn to risk assessment to try to manage and contain consumer volatility. If used in this way, it sets up a polarity between the expert – "we know best, don't worry your pretty little heads" – and the consumer (Wynne 1996). Treat people like children and they behave accordingly, quickly sensing victimhood (Gabriel & Lang 1955: 117ff).

There is a burgeoning literature on risk assessment and its application both in "hands on" and wider policy contexts (Wilson & Crouch 1987, Sapp et al. 1994, Sparks & Shepherd 1994). Companies specialize in risk control. Globally, in anticipation of the 1994 General Agreement on Tariffs and Trade (GATT), considerable thought was expended on thinking through its application in trade contexts (Codex Alimentarius Commission 1993).

Risk assessment is not without its critics. Some sociologists have argued that society is taking on a new cultural form, the so-called risk society where social institutions can no longer contain the risk that post-industrialization has engendered (Beck 1992). Science policy researchers argue that what is at stake is trust in institutions rather than risk itself and that excessive burden is placed on the victim to prove harm. Based on analysis of environmental crises such as Chernobyl (Wynne 1991), Wynne has argued that the "breakdown of trust is more to do with the inability of expert institutions to frankly admit ignorance, contingency and lack of control when appropriate, than with the supposed growth of risk *per se*" (Wynne 1996). Others suggest that risk assessment is a version of cost benefit analysis and acts as a mechanism of control (Adams 1996), substituting diverse, democratically accountable standards for harmonized standards imposed "top down" in the interests of large traders, rather than local small and medium enterprises (Avery & Lang 1993, Adams 1995).

Consumers' risk-reducing behavior: MAFF's own research

Despite this wider, theoretical debate about the role of risk assessment, the fact is that considerable research has been conducted on it. In 1993, MAFF was already considering the significance of consumers' perception of food-related risk. This work was addressing the importance of "assessing a risk tool-kit" for assessing consumers' perceptions "and taking them into account". The tool-kit was to include "improving communications about risk and formulating new policies". What has happened to this?

When choosing foods, studies have shown that even in low risk situations, consumers act to reduce risk (Mitchell & Boustani 1992). The dimensions of perceived risks include the physical, financial, emotional, social, and time. Such studies suggest that the Government's reliance upon science to inform consumers about risk was entirely inappropriate. Instead of meeting consumers half-way and addressing their concerns, Government advice was perceived as hectoring, irrelevant, inappropriate, and insensitive. This failure of management of risk communication is one of the more serious failings to be exposed by the BSE saga.

Uncertainties in the scientific process

And what of Government's own chosen area of evidence – the scientific advice much quoted by ministers over recent years?

The BSE crisis has been in the public arena for eight years. Since the disease became public in 1988, many Government reports have been written, parliamentary questions asked, conferences and reviews conducted (Department of Health & Ministry of Agriculture, Fisheries and Food 1989). The Commons Agriculture Select Committee reviewed the situation in 1990. MAFF has done an admirable job in updating the chronology of the disease (for example, Ministry of Agriculture, Fisheries and Food 1995). Not surprisingly, a positive torrent of press coverage was unleashed.

Large sums of taxpayers' money have been expended on an extensive monitoring exercise, and even more on the scientific endeavor to understand the etiology of the disease (Consultative Committee on Research into Spongiform Encephalopathies 1989). This effort has been driven by a concern to contain the epidemic and to prevent the disease jumping species to humans. Throughout the last six to eight years, a stream of reassurance from ministers and ministries was issued to the public to the effect that beef was entirely safe (for example MAFF 1990). Despite a number of public relations gaffs – notably by Mr Gummer when feeding a hot burger to his daughter – the message was unchanged: British beef is 100 per cent safe. The source of this assurance was said to be the scientists, but this is not the whole picture. Since the Southwood Report, caveats have been expressed in print. Even as recently as November 1995, MAFF was admitting to difficulties in "accuracy of clinical diagnosis" (MAFF 1995: 5).

Uncertainties were endemic in that a multiplicity of scientific disciplines all added insights.

Politicians, however, were more categorical than they ought to have been. Although Mr Gummer has taken most public flak, his predecessor is not without blame in this respect. John MacGregor, MP, then Minister of Agriculture, made a written reply to a question about Southwood which talks not of certainty, but of risk; the "risk of transmission of BSE to human appears remote and it is therefore most unlikely that BSE will have any implications for public health" (MAFF 1989: 1).

Mr Gummer, too, placed considerable faith on the categorical nature of science, arguing, for instance, against a ban on ruminant protein in pig and poultry feed thus: "Doctors and scientists see no need for that" (MAFF 1990: 2). He reiterated that Government policy was based on "the best independent scientific advice available", which is a mite more circumspect than the latter assertions that "beef is 100 per cent safe". By the mid-1990s, Government statements had banished any doubts, to a degree that was unwarranted (Pattison & Dealler 1995) and politically stupid. The Select Committee should ascertain why and how this transition occurred.

Management of the 20 March announcement
Although accusations about causes, conspiracies, and confusion have dogged BSE since its first appearance (Lacey 1994) nothing has been of the order or global reach that was unleashed once Stephen Dorrell, MP, the Secretary of State for Health, made the announcement on 20 March 1996 that there was a "possibility" that ten recent cases of Creutzfeldt–Jakob Disease might be due to BSE. The policy context changed dramatically, as did the tone and tenor of the discussion.

It is important to cite Mr Dorrell's exact words. He said that "a previously unrecognised and consistent disease pattern" had emerged, and despite their remaining "no scientific proof that bovine spongiform encephalopathy can be transmitted to man by beef, ... the Committee has concluded that the most likely explanation at present is that those cases are linked to exposure to BSE before the introduction of the specified bovine offal ban in 1989" (Hansard 20 March 1996: column 375). Statements from SEAC and the Chief Medical Officer on 20 March 1996 were similarly worded (see MAFF 1996).

The reaction to this announcement was considerable. So much so that the Secretary of State, Stephen Dorrell, joined with the Sun newspaper in the accusation that the public, not cows, were mad (BBC Radio 4, "Today", 26 March 1996). Yet no assessment of the Government's handling of this situation is worthwhile unless it accepts that public reaction to this momentous event was rational rather than irrational. Ministers might doubt public rationality, but such feelings were best kept private. By its own policy objective – the maintenance of beef sales – it was a disaster; sales halved, companies withdrew products, and a worldwide ban ensued.

Trying to woo consumers back: price and Euro-bashing

Because the Government was eight years into its strategy of maintaining beef while banning Specified Bovine Offal, the only mechanisms left to it were piecemeal. To retailers, the main mechanism was price. The triumphant announcement, first by J Sainsbury and then by Asda, that consumers had flooded back when induced by low beef prices were predictable. Consumers who wanted to eat beef would take advantage of bargains. The figures collected by the Irish Food Board give the lie to the assertion that confidence was back: the picture was, and is, more complex. Like many issues in contemporary consumerism, confidence was fragmenting. Some consumers had never lost it, some had never had it, some had had theirs weakened, and some were still making up their minds. The management of risk perception is itself a highly volatile entity.

Mixed messages about risk from BSE since 1989

For years Government had made what it is now suspected were unwarranted, categorical statements about beef being 100 per cent safe. Yet slightly different messages were also dispatched in the form of the gradual tightening up of regulations. Excellent chronologies of events have been published by MAFF (1995: appendix 1) and Professor Lacey (1994: xii–xv). From the consumers' point of view, messages were mixed: on the one hand, reassurance was being given about safety to an almost absurdly high degree, while, on the other hand, regulations about removal of specified bovine offal were being tightened up, thereby implying that perhaps they should have been tighter earlier. MAFF's own monitoring in 1995 underlined and contributed to this gap. Spot checks on abattoirs found a lamentable degree of failure to implement the Specified Bovine Offal (SBO) orders. The September check failed 48 per cent of establishments visited, and the October visit failed 34 per cent (MAFF 1995: appendix 3). It is anticipated that subsequent spot checks will show a better performance.

In trying to explain the slow response of the disease curve to the ban on specified bovine offal (Lacey: 127–8), MAFF has argued that "there has been some continued leakage of BSE infected material into animal feed" (MAFF 1995: 5). The spot checks seem to confirm this, but it is still unclear whether this explains the 25,000 animals which have gone down with BSE born after the SBO ban. Only the experiment MAFF is conducting into maternal transmission will begin to answer the other leading interpretation.

From the consumers' point of view, it has hardly been reassuring that throughout the BSE saga, MAFF's prognoses that the disease incidence would decline have had to be delayed. This predictive failure suggests that the etiology is not fully understood – hardly surprising in the face of such a new disease (Dealler 1996). Pronouncements of certainty should not be made in such circumstances, if they arise again.

MAFF and the Government continued to act and make pronouncements to the public as though they were in full control of the facts. To add insult to injury, the SBO spot checks suggest, not just a failure to enforce the SBO ban, but the morality and self-regulation of the feedstuffs industry.

The failure to enforce the SBO order raises questions about the validity of Mr Dorrell's 20 March statement that the ten CJD cases were linked to exposure in the period up to 1989. Exposure has probably been longer. Since early days, abattoir workers have complained about speed-up on the line, about the pressure to maintain a high throughput of carcasses. What is astonishing is, not that public reaction was so great from 20 March onwards, but why it was not greater from 1995 on.

Handling Europe and the world

When the 20 March announcement was made, the story went worldwide. The speed and scale of the dynamics intensified. The EC imposed a worldwide ban on UK beef exports, thereby killing off a prime export market which accounted for around 20 per cent of UK production. This action then engendered a furious counter-reaction from the Government and its backbenchers who argued, with some success, that this was an example of heavy-handed European bureaucracy; 55 per cent in the ICM poll agreed the EU was "over-reacting and being unfair" (Linton & Bates 1996). In a matter of days, a national public health issue became a site for a full-blown political show-down on a world scale. Beef consumption even fell dramatically in the rest of Europe.

According to figures from the Irish Food Board, consumption was down in the week of 15 April (compared to the period before Mr Dorrell's announcement on 20 March) by 45 per cent in Germany, 40 per cent in France and 30 per cent in Spain and Italy. In the UK, it was down by 36 per cent (Irish Food Board figures quoted in Southey (1996)).

Membership of Government's scientific committees

It could be argued that a better, more sensitive approach to consumers might have mitigated this dire effect. Only quick action in the early days of BSE (1988–89) could have retained public confidence in the Government. Instead, the Government displaced focus for action upon a tiny number of scientists. This strategy has now undermined science itself. How has this happened?

Over the last eight years, Government advice on BSE – at least that in the public arena – has been taken from three over-lapping committees: Southwood (a Working Party), Tyrrell (a Consultative Committee) (MAFF 1989), and SEAC (an Advisory Committee). The latter has been the key body under the chairmanship of Professor John Pattison since October 1995. Until a time coinciding with the appointment of Professor John Pattison, membership of these committees was drawn from too narrow a pool of expertise. In my submission to the 1990 Agriculture Committee inquiry, I argued that this was foolhardy, and that consumer representatives should be drawn into the deliberations (Agriculture Committee 1990); this did not happen.

The failure to include consumer and other representatives on key committees such as SEAC lies at the heart of the failure of Government since

1988. The membership of SEAC should be widened to include consumer, environmental health and social science expertise. Lessons should be learned across Government in this respect.

April 1996

References

Adams, J. 1995. *Cost benefit analysis. Part of the problem, not the solution.* Oxford: Green College Centre for Environmental Policy and Understanding.

Adams, J. 1996. *Risk*. London: University College London Press.

AGB Market Intelligence 1989. *Food scares: an assessment of the effect in the marketplace*. London: AGB.

Agriculture and Health Committees 1997. *Bovine spongiform encepalopathy (BSE) and Creutzfeldt–Jakob disease (CJD): report of hearings*. London: HMSO.

Agriculture Committee 1990. *Bovine spongiform encephalopathy (BSE)*. Fifth Report Session 1989–90. London: HMSO.

Avery, N., M. Drake, T. Lang 1993. *Cracking the Codex*. London: National Food Alliance.

Beck, U. 1992. *Risk society: towards a new modernity*. London: Sage.

Beveridge, W. 1928. *British food control*. Oxford: Clarindon Press.

Black, A. & M. Rayner 1992. *Just read the label*. London: HMSO.

Cannon, G. 1987. *The politics of food*. London: Century.

Clunies-Ross, T. & N. Hildyard 1992. *The politics of industrial agriculture*. London: Earthscan.

Codex Alimentarius Commission 1993. Risk assessment procedures used by the Codex Alimentarius Commission, and its subsidiary and advisory bodies. Report of a meeting, Geneva, 20th Session, 27 June–7 July. Rome: Codex Alimentarius Commission.

Consultative Committee on Research into Spongiform Encephalopathies 1989. *Interim Report, June*. London: Ministry of Agriculture, Fisheries and Food and Department of Health.

Consumers' Association 1991. *Consumers and Food Policy*. London: Consumers' Association.

Dealler, S. 1996. *Lethal legacy*. London: Bloomsbury.

Department of Health 1996. *Low income, food, nutrition and health: strategies for improvement*. London: Department of Health.

Department of Health & Ministry of Agriculture, Fisheries and Food 1989. Report of the working party on bovine spongiform encephalopathy. London: DoH/MAFF, February.

Department of Trade and Industry 1993. Press Release P/93/563, p. 1.

Dibbs, S. E. 1993. *Children: Advertisers Dream, Nutrition Nightmare?* London: National Food Alliance.

Fenelon, K. G. 1952. *Britain's food supplies.* London: Methuen.

Food Advisory Committee 1991. Food Advisory Committee Report on its Review of Food Labelling and Advertising 1990. FdAC/REP/10. London: HMSO.

Gabriel, Y. & T. Lang 1995. *The unmanageable consumer.* London: Sage.

Gajdusek, D. C. 1985. Subacute spongiform encephalopathies caused by unconventional viruses. In *Subviral pathogens of plants and animals: viroids and prions* K. Maramorosch & J. J. McKelvey (eds), 483–544. Orlando: Academic Press.

Genetics Forum 1996. Pulling off the confidence trick? *Splice of Life* 2(6), 6–7.

Gore, S. 1995. More than happenstance. Creutzfeldt–Jakob disease in farmers and young adults. *British Medical Journal* 311, 1416–18.

Grove-White, R., P. Macnaghten, S. Mayer, B. Wynne 1997. *Uncertain world: Genetically modified organisms, food and public attitudes in Britain.* Lancaster: Centre for the Study of Environmental Change, in association with Unilever.

Hammond, R. J. 1951. *Food: the growth of policy.* London: HMSO.

Hammond, R. J. 1956. *Food studies in administration and control.* London: HMSO.

Hammond, R. J. 1962. *Food studies in administration and control.* London: HMSO.

Jenkins, R. 1992. *Bringing Rio home, biodiversity in our food and farming.* London: SAFE Alliance.

Lacey, R. 1994. *Mad cow disease the history of BSE in Britain.* St Helier: Cypsela.

Lang, T. 1966. *The public health impact of globalisation of food trade.* Paper to 7th Public Health Forum. London School of Hygiene and Tropical Medicine, 1–3 April.

Lang, T. 1992. Food policy and public health. *Public Health* 106 (March).

Lang, T. 1995. The contradictions of food labeling policy. *Information Design Journal* 8(1), 3–16.

Lang. T., E. Millstone, H. Raven & M. Rayner 1996. *Modernising UK food policy: the case for reform of the Ministry of Agriculture, Fisheries and Food.* London: Centre for Food Policy, Thames Valley University.

Le Gros Clark, F. & R. M. Titmuss 1939. *Our food problem.* Harmondsworth: Penguin.

Leather, S. 1992. Less money, less choice: poverty and diet in the UK today. In *Your food, whose choice?* National Consumer Council, 72–94. London: HMSO.

Lees, A. and K. McVeigh 1988. *An investigation of pesticide pollution in drinking water.* London: Friends of the Earth.

Linton, M. & S. Bates 1996. Public suspects beef cover-up. *Guardian*, 3 April, p. 1.

Lobstein, T. 1996. Beef watch. *Food Magazine* 32, January, 6–7.

London Food Commission 1988. *Food adulteration.* London: Unwin Hyman.

Lupton, D. 1996. *Food, the body and the self.* London: Sage.

MAFF "Look at the label" Food Sense leaflet series. London: MAFF.

Ministry of Agriculture, Fisheries and Food 1989a. Consultative Committee set up to look at research into BSE and other spongiform encephalopathies. News Release 85/89. London: MAFF.

Ministry of Agriculture, Fisheries and Food 1989b. The Government's response to Southwood Report on BSE. News Release 84/89. London: MAFF.

Ministry of Agriculture, Fisheries and Food 1990. *BSE information pack.* London: MAFF Food Standards Division.

Ministry of Agriculture, Fisheries and Food 1995. *Bovine spongiform encephalopathy: a progress report.* London: MAFF, November.

Ministry of Agriculture, Fisheries and Food, Food Safety Directorate 1990. John Gummer's Statement on BSE. FSD 19/90. London: MAFF.

Ministry of Agriculture, Fisheries and Food, Food Safety Directorate 1993. Bulletin no. 41, September, p. 1–2.

Maynard, R. 1991. *Off the treadmill.* London: Friends of the Earth.

Miller, D. & J. Reilly 1994. Making an issue of food safety: the media, pressure groups and the public sphere. In *Eating agendas: food and nutrition as social problems* D. Maurer & J. Sobal (eds), 303–36. New York: Aldine de Gruyter.

Mills, M. 1992. *The politics of dietary change.* Aldershot: Dartmouth.

Mitchell, V. W. & P. Boustani 1992. Consumer risk perceptions in the breakfast cereal market. *British Food Journal*, **94**(4), 17–27.

Monopolies and Mergers Commission 1993. Animal Waste in England and Wales and in Scotland. Cm 2340. London: HMSO, September.

Monopolies and Mergers Commission 1991. Report on Prosper de Mulder Limited and the rendering business of Croda International PLC: a report on the merger situation. Cm 1611. London: HMSO, August.

National Consumers Council 1988. *Consumers and the Common Agricultural Policy.* London: HMSO.

Pattison, W. J. & S. Dealler 1995. Bovine spongiform encephalopathy and the public health. *Journal of Public Health Medicine* **17**(3), 261–8.

Paxton, A. 1994. *The food miles report.* London: SAFE Alliance.

Polkinghorne, J. 1994. Report of the Committee on the Ethics of Genetic Modification and Food Use. London: HMSO.

Raven, H. & T. Lang with C. Dumonteil 1995. *Off our trolleys? Food retailing and hypermarket economy.* London: Institute for Public Policy Research.

Roberts, R. W. 1995. Furrowed brow over mad cow. *British Medical Journal* **311**, 1419–20.

SAFE Alliance 1992. *What future?* London: SAFE Alliance.

Santer, J. 1997. Speech by Jacques Santer, President of the European Commission at the Debate in the European Parliament on the report into BSE by the Committee of Enquiry of the European Parliament, 18 February 1997. Speech 97/39.

Sapp, S., W. Harrod, L. Zhao 1994. Social construction of consumer risk assessments. *Journal of Consumer Studies and Home Economics* **18**, 97–106.

Southey, C. 1996. "German beef consumption falls by half". *Financial Times*, 23 April, p. 10.

Sparks, O. & R. Shepherd 1994. Public perceptions of the potential hazards associated with food production and food consumption and empirical study. *Risk Analysis* **14**(5), 799–806.

Tiemstra, J. 1992. Theories of regulation and the history of consumerism. *International Journal of Social Economics* **19**(6), 3–27.

Tracy, M. 1982. *Agriculture in Western Europe*. London: Granada.

Walker, C. & G. Cannon 1984. *The food scandal*. London: Century.

Wilson, R. & E. Crouch 1987. Risk assessment and comparisons: an introduction. *Science* **236**, 17 April, 267–70.

World Health Organization 1990. *Diet, Nutrition and the Prevention of Chronic Disease*. Technical Series, No. 797, Geneva: World Health Organization.

Wynne, B. 1991. Public perception and communication of risks: What do we know? *Journal of NIH Research* **3**, 65–71.

Wynne, B. 1996. Patronising Joe Public. *Times Higher Education Supplement*. 12 April, p. 13.

Chapter 7

Mad Cows and Englishmen

Ian Wylie

This chapter and the preceding chapter are based on talks given to the National Association of Health Authorities and Trusts (renamed NHS Confederation as of April 1997) and at St Catherine's College, Oxford, in the summer of 1996.

Seventy-three years ago, in a lecture in the small Swiss town of Dornach, the philosopher and teacher, Rudolf Steiner, posed the question: "What would happen if the ox were to eat meat directly instead of plants?" Steiner, who was an early advocate of organic farming, went on to propound to his Swiss audience his theory about unused energy in the animals' bodies and the consequent build up of harmful acids, which he thought would eventually attack the nervous system and ultimately the brain. This was not great science by modern standards, but his conclusion, in 1923, does have a modern ring to it. "If an ox were to consume meat directly," he ended, "the ox would go crazy" (Watts 1996: 17).

On 14 March 1996, the Chief Medical Officer of the UK, Sir Kenneth Calman, alerted the Secretary of State for Health, Rt. Hon. Stephen Dorrell, MP, that the Government's committee on mad cow disease, Spongiform Encephalopathy Advisory Committee (SEAC), was meeting to discuss notification from the disease control center in Edinburgh of 10 new cases of Creutzfeldt–Jakob's disease (CJD). The worrying thing about these new cases of CJD was that they occurred in young people, several of whom had had contact with the beef industry. The evidence of a possible link with bovine spongiform encephalopathy (BSE) was in direct contrast to the string of statements from both health and agriculture ministers and officials over the past six years that there was absolutely no link between the two diseases. Three days later, on Sunday 17 March, Stephen Dorrell was phoned at his home in Warwickshire, by his private secretary, to be told that SEAC had concluded that there may be a link between the new cases of CJD and BSE. "I was obviously very concerned," Dorrell said later to Jeremy Lawrence, *The Times* health correspondent, "but I was determined that we would proceed at a deliberate pace and not be seen either to be complacent or to over-react" (Lawrence 1996: 10).

The next day, Monday 18 March, Dorrell and Douglas Hogg, Secretary of State for Agriculture and Fisheries, briefed the Prime Minister. Professor John Pattison's expert committee, SEAC – or the Government Scientists, as they were to become known – were asked to draw up practical recommendations to tighten the controls governing animal feed and the processing of slaughtered cattle. SEAC met on Tuesday afternoon and deliberated until early on Wednesday morning, getting their recommendations to the regular Wednesday morning cabinet meeting. This meeting was attended by John Pattison and Kenneth Calman, who outlined the position and answered questions. The Cabinet then endorsed the recommendations. At 15:30 h the facts were given to the House of Commons in a statement by Stephen Dorrell and Douglas Hogg.

This could have been the end of it. Government finds cause for concern; Government takes expert advice and acts openly and quickly to make changes; public sees and hears decisive action; public is reassured. It could have been the end, but of course, it wasn't. Let me add two other things that happened in this first period. First, some of the cabinet, including, it was reported, Brian Mawhinney, the Conservative Party Chairman and former biomedical scientist, wanted to delay the announcement until SEAC had had more time to review the findings, and the Government had a more complete strategy. Dorrell opposed that, on the grounds that it would leak out anyway (as it had done that morning, led by the *Daily Mirror* headline "Official – Mad Cow Can Kill You") and that he was for open government, and the public's right to know. Secondly, even at the cabinet meeting there were questions that could not be answered. In particular, Gillian Shepherd, Education Secretary, was concerned about the implications for school pupils. How safe were our children? That cabinet disquiet spread to the House of Commons for Dorrell's ministerial statement: the House was full, suggesting that MPs' barometers were registering stormy weather ahead.

Why is this important for health communication? Well, let's examine what the public was hearing on Wednesday evening. First, the government's message was clear: "You know that for the last six years we have been telling you that there is absolutely no link between mad cow disease and the brain disease in humans, CJD, and that it is safe to eat beef. Well, there might be a link and it might not have been safe after all. In fact, you may already have eaten enough beef to give you degenerative brain disease, and so for that matter might your children."

Secondly, they were saying: "You know that for the last six years we have been telling you that even if there were a link between BSE and CJD (which of course there isn't), beef is safe because all the infected parts have been removed. Well, actually, we're not absolutely sure that they all have been removed, so we're introducing new measures which we hope will sort it."

And thirdly, they were saying: "The risks are so small that they are practically non-existent, so keep eating beef anyway."

The tactic that the Government took was the time-honored one: There is a public health alarm, and what the public needs is information, reassurance, and guidance. The Government attempted to provide these things, but by Wednesday evening, courtesy of the broadcast media, the public were getting thumbnail sketches of the history of BSE and the public decided that, in fact, they had quite enough information, thank you very much. In the UK and throughout the world, viewers took one look at past footage of Government experts swearing on their grandmothers' graves that beef was safe, and discounted them. Then the infamous television footage from 1990 of John Gummer, then Minister of Agriculture, giving a beefburger to his daughter was shown, and the viewership wondered how Ms Gummer's health was now, and people throughout Europe began to stop buying beef.

Now this seems to be the one thing that the Government hadn't expected to happen, and it was at this point, in the very first hours of the beef crisis, that ministers lost the picture. They thought, quite sincerely, that what was needed was more guidelines and information, reassurance by action, and openness. Dorrell recognized that the public would not necessarily trust the politicians, so he put his faith in scientists. Open government with nothing to hide would bind itself to their recommendations. Professor Pattison was asked to reconvene SEAC over the weekend to provide the country with answers to all its anxieties about beef and children.

But already things were moving by their own terrifying momentum. By Thursday evening, the effect of consumer choice was having a devastating effect on beef sales across Europe. Like financial markets, integrated European Commission (EC) markets collapse with frightening speed. The French were the first to ban British beef imports in a desperate but futile attempt to shore up consumer confidence in their own beef market. By Friday evening six other European countries had followed. The next day the decisive blow was delivered. Paul Preston, Chief Executive of McDonald's UK, announced that the burger chain was taking beefburgers off the menu in all 650 UK outlets. McDonald's had spent three days watching sales figures plummet across Europe, and now brilliantly seized the market initiatives by announcing that Big Macs would return on Thursday with non-British beef. A day later, Burger King, Wimpy and Wendy's, influenced by the market leader, had no alternative but to follow suit. On Monday, as SEAC concluded that eating beef derivatives was safe for babies and children, it was already too late. Later that day the EC imposed a worldwide ban on British beef. Disoriented by the total paralysis of an £11 billion industry in five days, Stephen Dorrell went on "Call Nick Ross" the next day and suggested that it was not the cows but the people that were mad (BBC Radio 4, 26 March 1996). The result was uproar. The Secretary of State for Health took pride in his Midlands retailing background, and experience in responding to markets and customer needs. His comment about mad people showed more than anything else the dilemma he was in.

Although this is the stuff of high political drama, the Government's response to the BSE problem does have some wider lessons for the way in which health care is provided in the UK. What seems clear from the beef crisis is that the Government was struggling to reconcile two modes of behavior. The first, which we might call the "partnership mode", was articulated by Stephen Dorrell to *The Times* health correspondent, shorter after the Nick Ross radio phone-in. It is the language of equality in the relationship between individual and state provider: "I am absolutely sure that in a modern democracy, the Government must trust the people, give them the facts, and leave them to draw mature conclusions" (Lawrence 1996: 10).

The second, in contrast, is the older "leadership model", which is summarized most famously in this quote from the 1930s: "In the case of nutrition and health, just as in the case of education, the gentlemen in Whitehall really do know better what is good for the people than the people know themselves" (Douglas Jay quoted in Timmins 1995: 101).

Why did the British Government get it so wrong? Well, the problem is that Dorrell's partnership model isn't really that at all, but merely a variant on the leadership model. The key is the word "mature". Presumably, if people can make mature decisions, they can, in Mr Dorrell's view, make immature decisions as well; but this is rather odd. No-one heard Paul Preston, the McDonald's boss, talking about his customers making mature or immature decisions about going in for a Big Mac. He didn't question whether they were making right or wrong decisions when they chose to stay away. In fact he said on the radio that weekend that he and his scientific colleagues at McDonald's thought British beef was safe, but that wasn't the issue.

Now getting the public involved in healthcare decisions is the largest issue in health communication at the present time. All other health communication issues take a back seat. But it is worth asking in what way the health service wishes to involve the public. Does the health service:

(a) Want to get the public to share in decisions?
(b) Want to get the public to share in mature decisions?
(c) Want to get the public to share in right decisions?

Health service managers don't talk about mature decision making, but about informed decision making. This idea sounds terribly reasonable, but it isn't. There's a world of difference between a decision based on information and an informed decision. Only the informed decision can be wrong, if it is decided that it was not an informed decision, or an ill-informed decision. So, if the public makes a decision that you, the expert, don't like, you are at liberty to say that they weren't in possession of all the facts – financial, managerial, operational, clinical, and so on. They were not able to exercise mature judgments. They did not come to an informed decision. It is a short step from saying that the public have made a factually incorrect decision to saying that they have made a morally incorrect decision. That sort of tactic has been used by dictators the world over to ignore the wishes of their people.

After the initial shock and before they started to blame Europe, the Government criticized the public for being ill-informed about the concept of risk and probability. Notice how "absolutely no risk", changes to "no measurable" or "no identifiable" risk. Thus, when Dorrell was asked on a BBC television program about BSE if he regretted saying that beef was safe, he replied no, because "beef consumption is in the normal meaning of the word safe" (*Panorama*, 22 July 1996). The argument against the stupid consumer becomes: "Even if there is a link between BSE and CJD, the chances of one individual being infected are about as rare as being knocked down crossing the road, say 1 in 250,000. As nobody has given up crossing the road on such odds, so it is irrational to stop eating beef. Therefore, nobody should give up beef."

This argument, however, completely fails to take into account how people use the notion of acceptable risk. I have to cross the road to go about my normal life and so the risk of being knocked down is something I have to live with. Therefore, 1 : 250,000 is acceptable. I can opt not to eat beef and still have a perfectly normal life: choosing to eat pork and so reduce my risk is highly rational. Therefore, 1 : 250,000 is unacceptable. People are very good at looking at relative loss and gain. Hence, when beef came back on the market at hugely reduced prices, the notion of a tradeoff was applied, and relative financial gain outweighed the risk so people bought beef again.

But the notion of trading off brings me to my central point for health. One of the big inroads made in health communication over the past few years has been public empowerment, and big steps have been taken. But rather than talk about empowerment, I think we should really be talking about disempowerment. Assuming a zero gain model, if someone gets power, the result is that someone else loses power. So if patients and the public are really to gain power, who is going to lose it? Politicians, clinicians, managers? Who is going to give it up? Surely we have to disempower the health service itself?

The mad cow crisis of 1996 is important for health because it crystallizes, in a few dramatic scenes, some central questions in the relationship between the health sector and the public. What is to be the basis of this relationship? If it is to be one of partnership, this must mean more than allowing the public to make decisions which have already been settled. It must mean being able to say that it is the people who must choose the values which underpin health care and who choose between competing priorities. And it is the legislators and the managers who must rediscover their roles as servants of the people.

References

Lawrence, Jeremy 27 March, 1996. Interview with Stephen Dorrell. *The Times*, p. 10.

Timmins, N. 1995. *The Five Giants: A Biography of the Welfare State*. London: Harper Collins.

Watts, Mark 31 March, 1996. The birth of BSE. *Independent on Sunday*, p. 17.

Chapter 8

BSE: A Tragedy is Public Health in Reverse

Dick Mayon-White

The typical tragedy goes from a hopeful situation to a disastrous ending. Public health should work in the opposite direction, starting with a bad event and moving towards a happy outcome, such as when the forces causing disease and suffering are overcome. This idea of looking at public health as a tragedy in reverse may help us to understand what has happened during the BSE (bovine spongiform encephalopathy) crisis from a public health practitioner's viewpoint. There are close similarities between public health and tragedies: both are about human endeavor, human weakness, and human suffering; both are public performances which are intended for audiences – and in modern times would not be funded without an audience; both are artificial, in the sense of being manmade, and yet both usually are influenced by natural forces; both are a subtle mixture of randomness ("luck"), and of inevitability ("fate" in tragedies, natural laws in medical science).

To analyze the public health response to BSE in Britain, we can consider the steps usually taken in public health responses to infection and then look at what has happened, and not happened, with BSE. Normally a public health issue starts with the observation of an increasing or excessive amount of disease (high incidence). This is typically reported as "an outbreak" or "an epidemic". The second step is to test whether the reports are accurate, and not due to a misdiagnosis or a misunderstanding of what is normal and what is an excess. Very rare diseases are often misdiagnosed. So-called outbreaks of common diseases are more likely to be a previous under-reporting; on the other hand, epidemics may be undetected for much the same reasons. When it is reasonably certain that there *is* a real increase in an infectious disease, lines of investigation are instigated to determine the source of the infection, the reasons for its spread, and the interventions that will control its spread or mitigate the effects of infection. Often control measures will be started before the cause and mode of spread are fully known. Precautionary interventions may be successful, or may appear to be successful if the outbreak comes naturally to an end. Control measures should be tested for efficacy by strictly independent reviews of outbreak management or by scientific application in subsequent outbreaks. Too often, control measures are not adequately tested but cannot be dismissed, and so they are added to the burdensome folklore of "what must be done" in the face of a threat of disease. The public and political leaders should insist on careful scientific evaluation with the same vigor as they demand precautionary actions. Science does not progress in a single straight direction. It is characterized by indirect moves, sometimes backwards, sometimes sideways, and always surrounded by uncertainty.

In the early phase of an outbreak, it is not unusual for there to be more theories of its cause than cases of human disease. It is typical that there are wide-ranging suggestions that the outbreak is due to factors such as industrial pollution, importation from abroad, governmental neglect, contamination by dirty neighbors, immoral behavior, conspiracies, poor education, mutant micro-organisms, or even invasions from outer space. Inevitably, nationalism, and political and commercial interests add further complexities to the theories. For the first ten years of the BSE epidemic, when there was no evidence of any increase in human disease, this multitude of opinion filled many hours of broadcasting and many columns of newsprint.

Veterinary and human medicine are practiced separately in Britain, and there are few opportunities for the exchange of knowledge between the professions. Most of the medical problems that occupy the time and attention of doctors are exclusively human in their nature and treatment. Most of the zoonoses (diseases transmissible from vertebrate animals to human beings) are medical curiosities, which rarely spread from person to person. Few doctors understand prion diseases, or expect to see a case. So it is not surprising that the medical profession in the UK should have been spectators rather than players in the BSE epidemic.

The recognition of 12 cases of a human disease, a new variant of Creutzfeldt–Jakob disease (CJD) that may be related to the BSE epidemic in cattle, has made it essential that we take stock of the public health actions to date. The earliest actions, in 1988, were to remove offal that might contain the BSE agent from human food supplies. Eight years on, this still appears to be the right policy although there is reasonable criticism of its execution, especially concerning the insufficient compensation to the meat industry for their losses and the inadequate supervision of the process. With hindsight, it appears that the Southwood Committee may have underestimated the risk of the BSE agent crossing the species barrier into human beings. In the context of the knowledge available at the time, the Southwood Committee's recommendations were a reasoned statement of the risks and possible precautions. Its successor, the Spongiform Encephalopathy Advisory Committee, has continued the scientific standards, giving a new and disturbing opinion in March 1996 that the first eight cases of the new variant of CJD could represent the human disease due to BSE.

The species barrier is an important concept in infectious disease epidemiology. Our hopes of eradicating some important infectious diseases, such as smallpox, poliomyelitis and measles depend on it. It explains why we are not plagued by the numerous infections that afflict other species, especially farm animals. However, no biological barriers are absolutely effective; the combination of high doses of infective material (or numerous exposures) with high susceptibility may result in human disease.

Whatever the validity of scientific opinions and government actions, I cannot escape the question of whether public health practitioners like myself should have acted differently. Until 1996, public health actions were very limited: the epidemiology of CJD was being studied by neurologists, who were best placed to diagnose it and to monitor its incidence; there were no human cases of spongiform encephalopathy that were directly linked to BSE, and the incidence of CJD in the UK was similar to the incidence of CJD in countries without BSE. The cattle disease, BSE, was being managed by the appropriate agency, Ministry of Agriculture, Fisheries and Food (MAFF). The public health role was to keep people informed of developments, and to try to ensure that the best expert advice was available and understood by the public. Clearly both scientific study and public health actions have to be conducted at a national level, because foodstuffs are distributed across the whole country so no area is exempt from risk. Yet we saw only some schools taking beef off the menu, and only some restaurants avoiding British beef – in 1996 – when the risk must have been higher eight years before. In the face of such silliness, concentrating on larger problems has much to commend it.

Today the challenges to the public's health are much greater than the single issue of BSE. Unfortunately, while it is possible that there will be hundreds of cases of the new variant of CJD, perhaps increasing the incidence of CJD by tenfold in the UK, the numbers will be small compared with other diseases of public health importance – such as lung cancer and HIV infection. The public health medical services in the UK are overstretched, trying to cover the commissioning of hospital care as well as the traditional areas of public health, such as the alleviation of poverty and inequality, the control of infection and diseases arising from pollution and poor housing, the promotion of healthier lifestyles, and good primary health care. So public health doctors must be certain that their time will be usefully spent before they take on new issues.

Another factor which weakens public health is the separation of local services into different agencies. Public health doctors are employed in health authorities, under the direction of the Department of Health and the NHS Executive. Environmental health officers who have the local responsibility for food safety are employed in local authority districts which are rarely the same as health districts. The areas covered by local representatives of MAFF, the Environment Agency and the Health and Safety Executive are also different. All these agencies may have their tasks and areas increased, often with a reduction in staff. Directives from various departments of central government pour down, regardless of local priorities. Although goodwill and common purpose overcome some of the difficulties, the present organization seems to be seriously ineffective for concerted action.

In taking up an issue, the tradition in public health has been to support the smaller or weaker parties. In the past this has been manifest in children's and women's health, or in confronting industry and landlords. In the BSE debate it is not easy to see who is the weaker party because the media and the consumers have enormous power, the farmers and food industry have strong allies, and the Government has access to the best information. Possibly, the health services are the weaker party, and the attention that public health doctors are giving to maintain them is in keeping with their traditions.

In modern times, when public health is a governmental service, medical opinions may be treated sceptically by the media and by critics of the Government. Although the public health doctors' independence is not safeguarded in the way that the original medical officers of health were protected, there is a strong ethic of speaking out on matters of importance. However, when there is substantial uncertainty about a health issue, outspokenness is an ineffective way of promoting understanding and influencing people to reduce risks.

The public health lessons from the BSE story are still emerging. The first is that events that seem scientifically improbable can rarely happen, and that we should be prepared to reverse our views and to act accordingly. So if and when we are sure that BSE has crossed the species barrier to humans, we must accept that this is a public health problem, not a veterinary one. Even if the number of cases does not rise far above the 12 possible cases now suspected, the responsibility for food safety should be changed to lie with a single government department which is exclusively committed to human health. The practice of public health, particularly the surveillance of new and increasing diseases that may be infections or may arise from environmental pollution, needs to be strengthened at the local level. Unless local public health functions are strengthened, central government bodies will lack the information on which to base sound national policies and be powerless to implement them. The history of public health shows that improvements occur with better organization and with technological advances. Time and technology will undoubtedly resolve the question of whether BSE has or can spread into the human population. Only better organization can reduce the harm and prevent similar problems.

Chapter 9

The Politics of BSE: Negotiating the Public's Health

Catherine Goethals, Scott C. Ratzan and Veronica Demko

> It is the duty of the prince to solve problems before public emotions
> make them unsolvable.
>
> (Machiavelli, *The Prince*)

BSE (bovine spongiform encephalopathy), known commonly as mad cow disease, occupied much of the European Union's (EU's) political agenda in 1996. Franz Fischler, European Commissioner for Agriculture, termed the BSE issue "the biggest crisis the European Union had ever had" (Southey 1996). Presently, the EU has determined there is incomplete scientific evidence to justify lifting the ban on British beef imports that was imposed on 26 March 1996. In mid-1996, the BSE issue was used as a tool to block other important matters, such as enlargement of the EU and the creation of a common currency at the intergovernmental conferences. Interwoven with the politics of BSE were fears of humans catching CJD (Creutzfeldt–Jakob disease) through the consumption of beef, threats of collapsing beef markets, and fragmentation pressures within the fledgling Union.

The main questions arising from the politics of BSE are the following:

(a) How could an issue that was scientific and medical in nature be used by several EU member states as a vehicle to show their political weight both on the homefront and within the Union?
(b) How did the main "players" use this issue to advance their own causes?
(c) Why did negotiations become divisive and not lead to better outcomes?

The mad cow issue quickly became a political battle, one that did not focus on the safety of public health, but rather on the protection of the beef market. From the outset, it was clear that the EU would be challenged to placate all parties concerned throughout the negotiation process. This was attributable partly to the complexity of the EU's composition (15 member states, each with different interests), as well as the fact that the matter fell under the competencies of Director General (DG) VI – Agriculture. This DG is one of the 24 within the European Commission (EC) that is central to the protection and efficient functioning of Europe's agricultural market, in which the beef market commands a major role. Also, the presence of strong agricultural lobby groups was an important factor in the protection of the multi-billion dollar beef industry.

An examination of the BSE crisis shows that no party involved acted objectively or independently. Even the "scientific" committees assigned to investigate the issue were subject to political pressures. Unlike true independent agencies that make decisions that affect public health policy and industry (such as the Food and Drug Administration in the US), the leadership entities in this case – the government officials of the UK and other EU member states – shifted constantly to accommodate political agendas.

This chapter focuses on the political activity in Europe in 1996. We discuss the BSE negotiations and how optimal applications of negotiation theory may have been helpful in reaching a timely and effective solution. While the authors recognize the limitations inherent in any theoretical application in such a complex issue, a retroactive study of the events in the BSE crisis may help to avert or avoid similar situations in the future.

The ideal of negotiation is based on a fundamental belief in the ethical responsibility of both the sender and the receiver of a message to participate actively in finding common ground and potential solutions to a shared exigence – defined by Bitzer (1968) as the perceived or real imperfection inviting a rhetorical response, and initially the indispensable condition for such an encounter. In this case, the exigence was an issue oriented at the national and international level, which affected the economy, science, leadership, and health. The defining characteristic of negotiation is that two or more people come together to participate and to discuss the causes and solutions of a jointly perceived exigence.

Despite the lack of a traditional negotiation table and of individuals defining themselves as "negotiators", a conflict resolution/shared decision-making model based on constant interactive communication among the participants can be useful in understanding the mad cow crisis.

In adopting a negotiation model, one can elicit ideal governance ideals espoused by Madison in the Federalist papers: "the cool and deliberate sense of community ought to prevail in government" (Hamilton et al. 1961: 384). Yet, such open and direct communication requires an active and interested public, with the ability to detect sham arguments and fallacious reasoning. An analysis of the messages that characterized the politics of BSE suggests that it has many components associated with negotiation. Effective leadership now requires a shared decision-making perspective, as government officials ideally should welcome each other's perspectives on vital issues and potential solutions to their nation's problems.

COAST – Communication, Options, Alternative Standards, Trust – is an approach to negotiation rooted in elements of Aristotle's classical views on rhetoric (Aristotle 1984). Accordingly, negotiation is a communication process based on shared similarities derived from ethical and caring relationships between people in pursuit of common goals. Its goal of identifying differences and facilitating optimal solutions among the alternatives is designed to forge the overall trusting relationship among participants necessary for long-term success in future encounters.

With communication as its core, COAST advocates constituents to be involved in the brainstorming of options, without judging viability or effectiveness during such a discussion. Through intensive communication encounters, the primary objective in this phase is to identify and to expand alternatives, agreed upon by the involved parties, that could be employed in reaching a common goal. Such alternatives are selected based on their suitability and agreement with specific standards – ethical, objective criteria sometimes defined by a credible third party. Eventually, trust, a major goal of COAST, is established through disclosure, reliability, and co-operation in a variety of encounters.

The degree to which trust exists between parties – a product of the frequency and quality of interactions – and the subsequent development of reciprocal images of character and trustworthiness serves as: (1) an indicator of the overall satisfaction of the encounter, and (2) a potential predictor of the support of programs and policies advocated by the participant (Deutsch 1958, 1973, Parsons 1963, Rotter 1971, Ajzen & Fishbein 1973, Riker 1974, Winter 1973). Building a relationship is the unquantifiable by-product of effective employment of COAST.

Ideally, following a COAST model involves a dialectical approach, replacing the unidirectional flow of public speeches between a government official and a passive public with a multidimensional interchange. It prods the journalist and commentator to be more active, not as an agenda setter, but as an ethical purveyor of substantive information necessary for erudite, participatory decision making.

Trust is vital to effective governance. Page & Shapiro (1992) write: "Ordinary citizens need not master the intricacies of policy analysis but can get the general drift by knowing whom to trust for a reliable conclusion – assuming, of course, that trustworthy cue givers are available." It is enhancing the degree of this trust within the relationship which COAST has as its goal. In a relationship characterized by trust among the parties, goals and objectives are jointly pursued with a certain amount of sacrifice expected (Osgood 1959, 1962, 1966).

As we opt for more meaningful rather than merely symbolic acts of communication in political decision making, designed to enhance our shared interests, a guiding principle must be the active participation of all parties, including the public, in the process. In the discussion that follows, we will track the politics of BSE through the main actors, the exigence, and the responses to the exigence, and we will explore the ways in which meaningful negotiation was or was not practiced at each stage of the crisis.

Actors

Germany

As the largest economic power in the Union, Germany was one of the main actors in the negotiation process of the BSE drama, promulgating BSE in media coverage. In 1995, German Health Minister H. Seehofer called for more objective reasoning on the mad cow issue. Yet, in January 1996 he intended to notify the EC of a regulation passed by the Bundesrat (German Parliament) calling for a ban on imports of cattle from the UK (*European Report* 1996f). This decision was the result of the detection of BSE on a German farm some time before, in a cow that allegedly came from Britain. Mr Seehofer was obliged to call for the ban because of the conflict that was created between the Bundesregierung (German Federal Government) and some of the Bundesländer (German Provinces), which stimulate both national independence and import restrictions. EC insiders initially believed that this threat of trade conflict was a bluff by Bonn to force the BSE argument into the open and they suggested that this German anti-UK beef lobby – aimed at protecting its own market – should be overcome once and for all.[1] Therefore, the EC intended to sanction Germany, stating that German leaders had not acted in compliance with the internal market regulations and that they broke EU rules on the free movement of goods.

EU officials defended the UK Government when it said that it had done everything in its power to reduce the dangers of infection which could arise from exports of cattle or beef products, and that it had acted according to the regulations that were laid down in 1986. However, the EC's defense of the UK did not make Germany change its mind. North-Rhine Westphalia Environment Minister B. Höhn, for example, claimed that: "British beef should not be on the market until it is quite clear that it represents no threat to public health" (*European Report* 1996a).

According to its official statements, the German government's only concern was public health. At this point we should ask ourselves if this was indeed the case or if the German authorities were acting in an attempt to protect their own beef market. The fact remains that repeated negative statements on the quality of British beef could not and did not have any positive influence on consumer confidence.

France

In France, fuel was added to the BSE debate when the French Medical Academy passed a unanimous resolution on 7 February 1996 calling for a ban on the sale for human consumption of certain types of tissue from bovine animals of British origin which were less than six months old. The Academy was also in favor of stepping up the monitoring of people at supposed high risk for CJD after three British farmers had died of the disease within a period of a year. The Academy added that although there was no proven link between BSE and CJD in humans, the public still had to be cautious.

The United Kingdom

Yet, it was not only Germany and France who made sure that BSE remained a topic of political discussion. The British Government's attitude is the primary force that led to the BSE crisis. This was due to three reasons. First, contrary to what the EU had claimed, the British Government had not sufficiently enforced the post-1986 regulations. It had not taken the proper precautions in slaughtering all animals in any particular herd in which BSE had been found, whereas other member states such as France and Ireland had done so. In not fully applying these regulations, the British Government betrayed the trust it had received from the EU. Secondly, the British decision to pay farmers only half the market price for infected cattle resulted in farmers rushing cattle to slaughterhouses where they were paid full price instead of half.

Finally, the UK Government's main political error was that British ministers emphatically insisted that BSE posed no danger at all to public health. In 1988, British Professor R. Lacey had pointed out the danger of the disease in cows. He also suggested that the disease could possibly be transmitted to humans. At that time, however, he had no definitive proof. Even though his view was shared by several scientists, the UK Government did not realize the magnitude of the reports and instead perpetuated a message that British beef was safe to eat.

The Exigence

On 20 March 1996, the UK's Advisory Committee on BSE published a report suggesting that there could be a possible, though not scientifically proven, link between BSE and CJD. It showed clearly that the British Government had indeed treated the BSE matter with laxity in order to protect its beef market. It also demonstrated that the UK could no longer abuse the trust of its European partners. Following the BSE report, the EC made arrangements to set up a Special Veterinary Committee (SVC). The task of the SVC was twofold: first, it was to examine the evidence presented by the UK and secondly, it was to advise the EU executive of any steps to take in order to safeguard public health against BSE.

But the formation of the SVC did not prevent some of the member states from taking the matter into their own hands. Germany and France reaffirmed their repeated warnings; the UK had damaged its credibility within the EU. First France, and then Belgium, decided to put a temporary ban on imports of UK beef; they were soon followed in their decision by the Netherlands, Portugal,

Sweden and Germany. The Chairman of the European Parliament's Consumer Protection Committee demanded action be taken in order to protect public health.

Although the trust the EU had initially given to the UK was weakened, an EC agriculture spokesperson stated that the 1986 rules (and especially the more stringent ones of 1990) had been properly implemented by the UK. In turn, the member states were required to comply with EU legislation on the free movement of goods. In giving the UK this credit, the EU put its own credibility at risk and provoked reactions from several member states. The Bavarian Minister for Agriculture, for example, accused the Commission of "neglecting its duty to protect the consumer". Regardless of the fact that BSE had initially been referred to as a matter of public health, the reactions of the continental member states became increasingly political.

The Response

This series of reactions led the UK to acknowledge that it had indeed made mistakes. The British Minister for Health Mr S. Dorrell, for example, promised to set up a £4.5 million research programme to look into the BSE–CJD connection and said that more stringent measures would be instated to monitor the slaughtering of cattle and the destruction of the entire UK cattle herd if scientific evidence could prove that this was necessary for public health. Despite the UK proposal, the EC decided to take stronger actions. Subsequently, on 26 March 1996, the European Agriculture Commissioner F. Fischler announced an EU-wide export ban on UK beef to calm consumers' fears. Meanwhile, UK authorities were asked to report on the measures put in place to control and eradicate BSE. Member states who had put a temporary unilateral ban on UK imports were asked to bring their national legislation in line with the new EU legislation. The announcement on the EU-wide export ban was evidently not welcomed by the UK, who questioned the Commission's competence to place member states' produce under a total export ban. The Commission ignored this argument. It claimed that the steps taken were necessary to prevent trade deflection – which falls under the scope of Article 115 of the EC Treaty. From this point forward, the negotiations between the UK and the EU could be described as a "cat and mouse game".

During the European Council of Ministers Deliberations of 2 April 1996, the UK Farm Minister Mr D. Hogg showed little willingness to make concessions without receiving promises that the export ban would soon be lifted. He did, however, announce the following measures: a ban on the sale of cattle over the age of 30 months; an outlaw of the use of protein meal from ruminants in feedstuffs; and a selective slaughter policy targeted at those herds found on larger farms that had experienced outbreaks of mad cow disease. But the drafted synthesis of the meetings indicates that the Ministers' main objective was "to restore consumer confidence in beef and beef products, stabilise ... the beef market ... and provide assurances to our trading partners" (*European Report* 1996b).

Thus the goal of both the EU and the UK was the same: not necessarily protecting public health, but restoring consumer confidence. This led principally to policy decisions regarding the trade ban, rather than on communication strategies for health; but there was disagreement as to how confidence should be achieved. On the one hand, the EU was convinced that improvement could be achieved through the measures being implemented by the UK. The UK on the other hand – primarily wanting its own market back – said that consumer confidence would be restored sooner if the ban were lifted earlier. However, much to Britain's dissatisfaction, the draft agreement of the Luxembourg Meeting did not include a lifting of the ban. Britain's reaction was that Mr D. Hogg refused to sign the ministerial accord. Still, the EU decided it would attach importance to the draft and that its final decision would depend on the findings of the SVC report. This report was due to be published six weeks later and would supposedly be the ultimate proof as to whether or not the ban should be lifted. On 10 April 1996, however, the SVC recommended the total ban stay in place and that there be no relaxation of the export restrictions on gelatine and tallow. EC officials feared that if there was no partial lifting of the ban, Britain would refuse to send a newly expected selective slaughter program to Brussels and that it would justify retaliatory bans against EU imports, which would inevitably lead to a deadlock.

One could ask if the reasoning of the SVC was more political than scientific. Indeed, in making "anti-British" statements, it decided to go against the advice of the WHO (World Health Organization) and a group of independent experts of the EC, who believed the ban was not justified since there was no proof of any link between BSE and CJD. Could it be that lobbyist groups of certain more powerful member states put pressure on what was supposed to be an "objective" committee? The decisions made by the SVC seemed to be based, not on the severity of BSE among cattle, nor on exploring the possible link between cattle and humans, but rather on political compromises and the protection of beef markets.

Fortunately, the disputes did not lead to a deadlock. The UK Government designed its own plan for the disposal of cattle that adhered to the anti-BSE measures demanded by the EU. The UK also seemed willing to work out a plan that was designed to accelerate the eradication of the disease among UK herds, in order to achieve a lifting of the temporary import ban on all UK beef products and derivatives. It was also announced that the UK Agriculture Minister would co-operate with DG VI. Given these "concessions", one could have expected the EU to do anything in its power to come to a resolution. Nothing, however, could be less true.

After Britain had finally shown some willingness to solve the matter, a statement was made by Mr Fischler that: "the purpose of the beef export plan was to protect Europe's markets abroad" and that it was "safe to eat British beef" (*European Report* 1996c). This statement was rather unfortunate because it seemed to indicate that the ordeal around the BSE issue was exaggerated and that Britain had been unduly sanctioned. It also showed that the ban was in place not for safety reasons but rather to restore market confidence in EU beef products. The subsequent and well-known threat of the UK to bring the matter before the European Court of Justice was not welcomed. Mr M. Rifkind, Secretary of Foreign Affairs, spoke of "undesirable implications"[2] for the Union if the ban stayed, referring to a possible wielding of the UK's veto right to paralyse Union business or to refuse payments to the EU's budget. Still, new talks occurred between Mr Fischler and Mr Hogg in view of the EU Agricultural Meeting of 29/30 April 1996 in Luxembourg. In Brussels, intense speculation continued as to what concessions Hogg could expect from Fischler in arriving at a partial slaughter plan, since the former had ruled out all plans to slaughter the entire herd.

A UK Proposal

By 1 May 1996 both the Commission and Mr Fischler were impressed by the 40-page report submitted by the UK. It was referred to as a "logical, rational and sole model that could be used for further discussion" (*European Report* 1996e). In return, Mr Fischler promised to prepare outline strategies for the Council Meeting of 20 May 1996 and he reported to the SVC that, according to WHO guidelines, gelatine and tallow were perfectly safe for human beings and that semen represented no risk. The UK attempted to convince the public that efforts were underway to speed up the eradication of BSE. Both Fischler and Hogg had the same interest at heart: trying to arrive at a solution of the dispute and in so doing, restoring consumer confidence. Unfortunately, this shared agenda as the basis of negotiations was doomed to failure since it overlooked the cause of the exigence: a disease that was feared to be spread to humans. Negotiations still overlooked the health implications and focused instead on economic implications.

Britain promised that a plan was under way to remove older cattle from the food chain. The pressure Major was under in his own country was enormous. In view of the upcoming spring elections – already termed "beef elections" – he found himself caught between two opposing parties. On one side there were the retaliators, or the Euro-sceptics, in favor of sanctioning the EU and pursuing the empty chair policy at EU negotiations; i.e. their absence during negotiations would inevitably lead to a veto situation when voting was required. On the other side, there were the conciliators led by Mr M. Hesseltine, in favour of more "peaceful" negotiation strategies.

Despite positive reactions from ministers on the talks between Hogg and Fischler, Germany and Austria were still wary of any attempt to lift the ban. The input of other member states, who, like the UK, seemed more interested in protecting their own economy than in protecting public health, led to repeated deadlocks. The agreed agenda between Fischler and Hogg – restoring consumer confidence and solving the dispute – was entirely different from the one the member states had in mind – protecting their own beef market. Subsequently, among the members of the EU there were no shared interests and no room was made to discuss further possible options or alternatives.

During the European Council of Ministers Meeting in Luxembourg on 30 April 1996, the EU veterinary officers revealed their role in a delicate political process by calling for stronger measures. This required that a lifting of the ban would not take place too early, in order to satisfy public opinion that real action was indeed taken to ensure beef was safe to eat and to protect consumers against any risk of contracting CJD through the food chain. On 11 May 1996 it seemed obvious there would at least be a partial lifting of the ban on gelatine products, thanks to the persistent efforts of Mr Fischler.

Fischler's proposal to stop the ban on gelatine, tallow, and semen was rejected by the SVC on 20 May 1996. Following these developments, Major announced he would disrupt EU day-to-day business. Moreover, the results of the 3–4 June meeting led to frustration, since the UK wanted a definite framework for the progressive lifting of the ban. Once again, the agendas of the involved parties varied and there was the danger that the communication would seriously be damaged. The Commission and some of the member states firmly believed that it was impossible to get to a precise framework and that the UK Government should finally start to see the whole process as a trade; i.e. the EU would give in if necessary measures and controls were in place. The UK stated that it was willing to embark upon a targeted cattle slaughter plan, provided there were some assurances that this would lead to a direct lifting of the embargo. Both the UK and the EU appeared willing to look for possible options in order to avoid a new deadlock situation.

Tactics

However, when Major threatened to disrupt the EU's day-to-day business it was not a bluff. Tensions rose when the UK decided to start its non-cooperation procedure because of the refusal of the SVC to come to a partial lifting of the ban. One of the UK government's first retaliatory actions was the veto it put on the opening of EU trade negotiations with Mexico, which seriously damaged Spain. In its turn, Spain threatened to react if a Britain-backed trade agreement was signed, knowing the importance Britain attached to the application to entrance of certain central European countries to the EU. In keeping with negotiation theory, rather than playing this "tit-for-tat" game, Britain could have looked for options to bring the parties closer together. There was no longer a shared agenda and there was little willingness to search for possible options.

Major's tactics were under criticism both from the EU and the EP (European Parliament). Consumer Policy Commissioner, Mrs E. Bonnino, for example, said: "Everybody has their own methods and tactics, but this is not an appropriate negotiation strategy. We must not begin a built-up confrontation"

(*European Report* 1996e). Her view was shared by almost all EU partners. On 23 May 1996 a disappointed Fischler stated in an Austrian newspaper interview that the British attitude was "anything but useful" and that "The Government in London is giving the impression of putting its domestic political problems before consumer rights". One of the Belgian diplomats who had been involved in the negotiations on the revision of the Maastricht Treaty expressed his disappointment by saying that before the Brits had basically accepted anything and now they blocked everything (Boval 1996).

The UK decision to bring the matter before the ECJ led Commission President Mr J. Santer to state on a BBC television program *On the Record* on 26 May 1996 that the UK Government had been guilty of "mismanaging" the whole affair and that Major's non-cooperation procedure would not help to restore consumer confidence. He pointed out that this strategy was counter-productive and that he feared increasing anti-British attitudes among other member states, which in turn would lead to an even stronger isolation of Britain. In another interview, he said it was very unfortunate that Major was using the European issue as a means of bringing a truce between the warring Eurofractions in his Conservative Party, to whom he wanted to profile himself as a "master strategist". The evolution of the negotiations, from which no positive elements had emerged in Britain's favor as yet, indicated that he was not a master strategist at all.

During the Farm Council Meeting of 3–4 June 1996, British leaders indicated that they would only be willing to stop their non-cooperation policy on two conditions. First, the ban on beef derivatives should be lifted, and secondly, the promise had to be made that the entire beef embargo would be lifted progressively. Since Major insisted that any targeted cattle slaughter plan would be implemented in the context of a definite framework for lifting the ban, the feared deadlock arrived. Six countries opposed the proposal, including Germany, Austria, Portugal and the Benelux. From this moment, the whole UK strategy tended towards overt political lobbying, especially since Hogg had failed to impress and convince other member states of the safety of beef through factual presentations of anti-BSE measures.

Even though the Commission took an in-principle decision on 5 June 1996 to lift the UK derivative ban, the basis for a "framework" agreement still remained unclear. The UK authorities continued to press for an agreed "framework" for an overall lifting of the ban; something which would be very difficult to achieve. However, despite strong resistance from Germany towards political compromise with the UK and the continued pressure from the SVC on London to widen the scope of its plans to eradicate BSE from its national herds, ministers came close to agreement on the framework plan to end the UK ban. These efforts and concessions were made in view of the coming Intergovernmental Conference (IGC) in Florence where important matters, such as the Monetary Union, were on the agenda.

The UK agreed to trace BSE-infected animals born between October 1990 and June 1993 to their original herds and then further trace and destroy cattle of the same age. This re-thinking of the slaughter plan was a result of the latest statistical evidence that existing controls on animal feed would cause BSE to die out in the UK within four to five years even without the proposed targeted cull of "cohorts" of all infected cattle born between 1989 and 1993. At the request of the SVC, the UK agreed to extend this scheme to animals born between 1989 and 1990, but only if such actions would prove to be "scientifically justifiable". The stumbling block to the framework agreement was that the UK wanted a freeing of exports to certain third countries. The main argument linked to this request was that UK consumers were still eating British beef, thus there was no legal justification for a ban on third countries not authorised to export meat back to the Community.

During the IGC at Florence the EU backed the "framework" plan for lifting the ban, thereby putting an end to the non-cooperation procedure and allowing Major his "face-saving" compromise. This did not imply, however, that the matter was entirely removed from the political agenda. Major's optimism about having the entire ban lifted before the end of 1996 would prove to be wishful thinking. Proceedings at the Florence Summit caused the public to react against the political slant the issue had acquired over the past months. The fact that a public health issue was dealt with as a purely political matter led to heavy criticism. During the Parliamentary Hearing of 24–25 June, for example, European Consumer Organization Director Mr J. Murray, was highly critical when he stated:

> Obviously, human health is of paramount importance and decisions must be based on scientific evidence and not on political horseriding. ... Policy-makers must also take into account what consumers want if consumer confidence is to be restored. Consumers have lost their confidence not only in beef but also in official authorities and feel excluded from the decision-making process. (*European Report* 1996d).

Mr Murray's statement indicated that what had begun as negotiations on the protection of public health ended up as negotiations on how to protect the member states' beef markets. Also, the more politicians bickered, the more panic was created among European consumers, and the less faith the public had in the handling of the situation. Communication – whether good or bad – had taken place but without taking into consideration a key partner: the consumer. This group had not sufficiently been involved in the process of looking for solutions. Maybe if they had, other alternatives would have been generated. This could have been achieved if the goal of all negotiations had centered on health. In this case, an independent and unbiased inquiry could have been performed as the basis for policy decisions. Even the simple measurement of public opinion and concerns regarding BSE could help determine a political communication strategy. This could be achieved with social scientific measurements (i.e. polling, focus groups, etc.) as well as personal meetings with associations, citizens, and labor groups.

Those who believed that the "agreement" reached in Florence would soon end the bickering over BSE were wrong. By mid-September the UK Government was determined to re-open discussions with their EC and EU partners on plans to slaughter thousands of cattle most at risk from BSE in order to achieve an entire lifting of the ban. This British determination was likely to weaken the prospects of lifting the ban on UK beef exports and could lead to putting into question compensation payments for British farmers from Community funds. Moreover, by 13 September 1996 there had not yet been notification from London on proposed changes to the slaughter program, which was contrary to the agreement in Florence on arriving at an eventual lifting of the ban.

Meanwhile, unilateral measures by the member states continued. France and Spain had banned the import of all meat and bonemeal products from all countries seen as being at risk from BSE. During a BBC television interview in September, EC President Mr J. Santer said: "It is not a good idea to have BSE back in the news every fortnight if we want to restore consumer confidence. The UK should stick to the Florence plan."

Mr Fischler warned the UK that if it did not carry out the selective cattle slaughter – following the Anderson Report (1996) and the report from the Spongiform Encephalopathy Advisory Committee – the possibility of lifting the ban would be seriously endangered.

As had been the case in the Florence Summit, strong efforts were made to keep the BSE issue off the Dublin Summit Agenda. The Florence framework, constructed by the EU Heads of State and Government, was essential for the continuation of positive talks. In order to discover scientific proof, the EU SVC and the Multi-Disciplinary Committee on BSE were studying two reports. The framework provided a ban on the mammal and bonemeal (MBM) feed considered by some to be responsible for the spreading of BSE, a selective cull designed to target cattle that had eaten the contaminated MBM, and the institution of improved cattle identification systems. The mad cow issue had progressed so that most people assumed that if cattle ate MBM, that was how cows got the disease, and hence if people ate cows, people could contract CJD.

Conclusions

Today, the BSE issue is still far from being solved. Presently, no agreement has been reached on an entire lifting of the ban or appropriate strategies to avert similar crises in the future. Although the matter turned out to be an expensive experience both for the EU and the UK, with $28 billion spent by the European Union in subsidies to the beef industry alone (Butler 1997), some lessons can be drawn from it. Hopefully these lessons will prevent a repeat of the way the issue has been handled, and will help leaders negotiate more effectively about future issues.

(a) The British attitude in the initial phases of the BSE crisis determined the complexity of the negotiation process. The laxity with which the UK treated the matter led to serious repercussions. The UK should have implemented the post-1986 regulations with proper documentation. This would have built some trust in government activity that it had listened to, and acted upon, repeated scientific advice in a reliable fashion. Moreover, the British Government could have provided more financial means to perform scientific research. During the crisis, Mr Major used BSE to strengthen his own image to the Euroskeptics in his own party.

(b) Britain, as well as other member states were guilty of using their veto right, not only having the power to sabotage other member states' trade and day-to-day business, but also obstructing the Union's future with regard to the accession of central and eastern European countries. The BSE incident suggests that the EU's institutions and decision-making mechanism are not ideal for 15 member states. Institutional reform must begin, including elimination of the tyranny of the veto right. The EU also needs a stronger Commission, because only it can preserve unity. In order to do so, however, a practical approach needs to be found that combines representativeness with efficiency. Finally, until this day the European Parliament still has no right to co-decide[3] on agricultural affairs. Article 43 of the EC Treaty provides for consultation, not for co-decision powers. Therefore, this section of the Treaty should be modified so that Parliament can function as the watchdog for the European citizens' interests. Legitimacy should come from the Parliament, not from the Council.

(c) The European political environment focused on policy rather than research. Some scientists had been claiming since the 1980s that they wanted to conduct research on a possible link between BSE and CJD. The number of permanent medical/health advisors as well as those in strategic communication in the Commission is very low and should be increased. More independent committees consisting of scientists should be established with new regulations that allow for active involvement of scientists in political discussions on scientific affairs. Moreover, scientific advice should be given by scientists and not by politicians. At the very least, if politicians insist on issuing advice, they should be guided by scientists. Government actions in the BSE crisis turned what should have been a medical/health problem into a political one.

The EU must begin to revise the CAP (Common Agricultural Policy) as far as research is concerned. Research of BSE is symptomatic of the CAP research program in general. Why would the EU not be able to adopt the same policy on scientific research as the US does? Public health should not be a tool in a battle of political dominance, nor should scientific evidence or real dangers to public health be compromised by personal and national political ambitions. One potential solution to this dilemma is the establishment of a permanent, objective food and drug agency which would operate on a system similar to the FDA in the United States. While it would not solve all food safety issues, it could serve as an independent scientific agency, if established with minimal political or industrial ties.

(d) The BSE crisis illustrates that the Union cannot return to protectionism and fragmentation. All member states of the Union have to realize that co-operation is the key to ensuring the future of an effective European Union. The BSE issue clearly showed that there is still a danger of member states trying to protect their own markets, despite the legal provisions on the free movement of goods. Britain cannot do without "Europe" because of its trade within the EU's single market and the foreign investments that come with EU membership. At the same time, "Europe" cannot do without the UK, because of the size of its market. To be successful in the changing global environment, member states should not let issues like mad cow disease threaten the unity of European States.

(e) The potential for negotiation and dispute resolution of the mad cow issue in a judicious manner required expedient decision making and leadership. Just as the COAST model suggests, establishing an agenda while focusing on interests and identifying key players was paramount. Further, establishing ground rules of who had authority to speak and make decisions would have helped all parties to articulate a consistent message. Instead, players had different interests, which led to debate and conflicting media messages. Leadership interested in serving the public and assuring the conditions so that the best decisions can be made, ought to approach future cases as negotiation, with fortitude and speed.

Summary

In an era of European expansion and changes in the European Union, new approaches with effective decision making in governance must be encouraged. New European politicians must possess a uniquely balanced perspective, based in ethical communication, with the ability to discriminate among values, craft effective messages to different audiences, and to negotiate with the best interests of the public in mind. In addition, new European politicians must exemplify the appropriate leadership abilities, credibility, and consensus building necessary to gain support for their policies. COAST centers on what unites us, not what divides us. It beckons each of us to apply realistic standards which benefit what we determine to be the public good. Its beginning is communication; its end is trust. COAST relies on the character of each one of us as its ethical engine, moving us toward effective governance in the days, months and years ahead.

Notes

1 Much of the information in this chapter comes from corroborating personal interviews with government officials who wish to remain unnamed.

2 Council Deliberations at EU Foreign Ministers Meeting, Luxembourg, 22 April 1996.
3 The co-decision procedure was reinforced by the Maastricht Treaty and entails the following concept: proposals by the Commission must be accepted by the Council. However, the parliament has the right to amend proposed texts and send them back to the Commission. The Commission then returns the proposal to the parliament, but if the parliament refuses a proposal twice, the procedure stops without having sent the text to the Council.

References

Ajzen, I. & M. Fishbein 1970. The prediction of behavior from attitudinal and normative variables. *Journal of Experimental Social Psychology* **6**, 466–87.

Anderson report 1996. Position statement of 29 October 1996 of the Institute of Food Science & Technology. Section: Current hot topics article: "Bovine spongiform encephalopathy (BSE)". Parts 1/3 and 2/3. 22 November 1996, pp 5–6.

Aristotle 1984. *Rhetoric*. London: William Heinneman.

Bitzer, L. 1968. The rhetorical situation. *Philosophy and Rhetoric* **1**, 1–6.

Boval, C. 1996. Gekke koeien verstoren (eu) forie. *De Standaard Magazine* 27 December: 15.

Butler, D. 1997. Science advice, a year of dangerous living: How BSE crisis forced Europe out of its complacency. *Nature* **385**, 6.

Deutsch, M. 1958. Trust and suspicion. *Journal of Conflict Resolution* **2**, 265–79.

Deutsch, M. 1973. *The resolution of conflict: constructive and destructive processes*. New Haven, Connecticut: Yale University Press.

European Report 1996a. Animal and public health: Commission to re-examine the evidence on UK mad cow disease. 10 February: 2106.

European Report 1996b. Farm Council: ministers burn the midnight tallow over UK beef ban. 3 April: 7.

European Report 1996c. Internal Market, Animal and Public Health: UK farmers consider legal action against beef export ban. 17 April: 5.

European Report 1996d. Internal Market, Mad Cow Disease: The crisis is far from over. 26 June: 8.

European Report 1996e. Internal Market, Mad Cow Disease: UK arguments impress commission and farm ministers. 1 May: 12.

European Report 1996f. Internal Market: UK takes the European Union hostage. 25 May: 12.

European Report 1996g. Veterinary policy: Commission considers actions against German ban on UK cattle. 19 January: 487.

Hamilton, A., J. Madison & J. Jay 1961. The cool and deliberate sense of community ought to prevail in government. In *The Federalist Papers*, C.

Rossiter (ed.), No. 63, 384. New York: New American Library.

Osgood, C. 1959. Suggestions for winning the real war with communism. *Journal of Conflict Resolution* **3**, 295–325.

Osgood, C. 1962. *An alternative to war or surrender.* Urbana, Illinois: University of Illinois Press.

Osgood, C. 1966. *Perspective in foreign policy.* Palo Alto, California: Pacific Books.

Page, B. & R. Shapiro 1992. *The rational public.* Chicago: University of Chicago Press.

Parsons, T. 1963. On the concept of influence. *Public Opinion Quarterly* **27**, 37–62.

Riker, W. H. 1974. The nature of trust. In *Perspectives on social power*, J. T. Tedeschi (ed.). Chicago: Aldine.

Rotter, J. B. 1971. Generalized expectancies for interpersonal trust. *American Psychologist* **26**, 443–52.

Southey, C. 1996. Fischler attacks UK for scrapping cull deal. *Financial Times* 24 September, 1996: 2.

Winter, D. G. 1973. *The power motive.* New York: Free Press.

Chapter 10

Protecting Health: Can the UK do Better?

Simon Hughes

The BSE (bovine spongiform encephalopathy) crisis of 1996, and subsequent developments, has raised many questions about the way health-related stories are transmitted to the public, the way governments treat citizens in the dissemination of information, and, especially, the trust between governors and governed in the formulation of public policy. Few may be blameless in the events and missed opportunities that led up to the explosion of concern in the media about the safety of meat, which many quite rightly continue to eat with negligible risk to their health. But the biggest culprit is undoubtedly the Government system that allowed BSE to become an issue of huge national and international importance, devastating the lives and livelihoods of thousands of farmers, producers, and sellers. The central irony should not be lost: the system that is skewed so obviously towards the interests of the producers – and more importantly was perceived to be so – was the direct cause of the grief meted out to those very people.

The Government originally implied that British beef does not place those eating it at risk of BSE. Later the careful wording of official statements, the withdrawal of British beef from school menus, and the statements by senior scientists that they would no longer eat British beef, suggested that the "powers that be" knew far more than the British people will ever know. One British scientist who had suggested that there might be a risk to human health after eating BSE-infected meat was labeled "evil" by the establishment. This is no way for the Government of a so-called civilized nation to behave when the very lives of its citizens are at risk.

The research into BSE has been carried out in a quite extraordinarily centralized and secretive way. The MAFF (Ministry of Agriculture, Fisheries and Food) owns all of the bodies of cows infected with BSE, and controls all of the epidemiological data. It has been exceedingly difficult and often impossible for scientists outside MAFF to get hold of tissue samples or data. Only one outside group (at the University of Oxford) has been allowed to analyse MAFF's data, and then has had to seek permission from MAFF before revealing any results. If the data had been released five years earlier, the culling strategy might have helpfully reduced the impact of the epidemic. Meanwhile, during 1996 MAFF had an exclusive agreement with Electrophoretics International (chaired by a

Conservative MP) to develop a diagnostic test for BSE. It is impossible to find out the exact agreement with Electrophoretics (why?), but there is no doubt that its exclusivity hindered the progress of many other companies from commercializing a test for BSE.

The BSE affair has overturned a can of worms, which squirm only partly because of the Government mishandling of the nation's health and cattle herds. At present, in Britain's uncodified constitution, ministers are accountable to Parliament, civil servants are accountable to ministers, and the public right to know is hedged around by no fewer than 250 secrecy provisions in various Acts of Parliament. Aside from limited statutory rights, there is no general right for the public to know what the Government knows. The first question has to be why we do not follow the example of other developed countries and put the responsibility on Government to justify secrecy, instead of on the public to justify access.

Citizens, Consumers, or Subjects?

A recent countrywide survey found that three-quarters of people felt it was difficult to know whether government advice was free from political pressures. In fact the Government was less trusted than even the food industry! Is it any wonder that when Douglas Hogg, as Minister of Agriculture, tells people that beef is safe, they instinctively err on the side of unbelief? One is reminded of the original BSE scare, several years ago, when a Government minister fed a beefburger to his five-year-old daughter in front of the inevitable media circus, to try to prove that beef was safe. Any credible co-ordination between politics and public safety has been destroyed, and has yet to be redrawn. Consumers need to have confidence that their interests are represented in Government policy.

The next question is how a ministry that, in its own words, laudably aims to "improve the economic performance of the agriculture, fishing and food industries" can possibly expect to be trusted when reassuring consumers about the safety of products that it is there to protect? When MAFF openly admits it is there to protect the food industries, it is the shopper on the street who has to avoid the BSE- and *E.-coli*-infected beef, the salmonella-infested eggs, and the cheese crawling with listeria. Consumer interests are diffuse and thinly represented, compared to the well-financed and well-organized producer interest groups. Special efforts, therefore, are needed to involve consumers at all levels of decision making.

At the very least there is a need for informed consumer representation on the specialist committees which serve and inform both the Department of Health and MAFF on food safety issues – committees such as COMA (Committee on Medical Aspects of Food Policy), ACNFP (Advisory Committee on Novel Foods and Processes), ACMSF (Advisory Committee on the Microbiological Safety of Food), SEAC (Spongiform Encephalopathy Advisory Committee), COT

(Committee on the Toxicity of Chemicals in Food, Consumer Products and Environment) and FAC (Food Advisory Committee). Such representation would lead to public scrutiny of information considered by the committees, which could well help restore the lack of confidence in government. Proposals to Government about action and research need to be systematically acted upon and reviewed and we must end the disproportionate influence held by the food industry on these committees.

The UK has no explicit national food policy, so by default we have a bad food policy. One's diet plays a crucial role in one's health and well-being. The incidence of heart disease in the UK is high, and this fact along with the countless food scares hurled at the British public suggests that consumers need to be adequately and reliably informed about what constitutes a healthy diet, and how to achieve it. It is necessary that people have easy access to foods which make up a healthy diet. To achieve this, there is a need for a strategic, co-ordinated approach to food production, food processing, consumer education and information in line with identified aims and objectives centered on public health.

A Food Agency

There is also a growing need to provide a focus, and clarify and co-ordinate responsibility, for all food issues in Government. This also extends to information provided by the Government. At the moment public announcements, campaigns, and information provided in leaflets and packs are not consistent or co-ordinated. On occasion, this inconsistency borders on the bizarre – for example when the Department of Health was working to reduce fat intake whilst, at the same time, a rather rotund MAFF Minister was judging the "Fish and Chip Shop of the Year Competition". An independent food agency could provide authoritative advice and support to Government. The agency could work at arm's length from the Government, free from day-to-day political pressures – a step which is urgently needed – but would investigate, report and monitor food policy. This body would work across Government departments, to ensure a consistent approach. It would co-ordinate data collection, and monitor services, surveillance and enforcement, and hold this information centrally.

Such an agency could have its activities co-ordinated by a council of independent experts, bringing with them knowledge of nutrition, micro-biological safety, food technology, toxicology, and food law enforcement. To maintain independence, members of the council would receive no funding from food producers; and any involvement in political or commercial interests, including earlier research funding, would have to be declared. There would also be a balance of consumer and producer representation.

Information from the agency would be communicated in a clear and independent way, published independently from the Government. Committees which advise Government departments would report to the agency, which would then publish conclusions and findings. Among other powers, it would plot food safety, dietary and nutrition trends, monitor the enforcement of legislation, and publicize deficiencies.

If such an agency comes into existence, consumer confidence in Government food policy can only improve; closer co-operation between Government departments, and a clear public health agenda, would result. Without such an agency, confidence will remain at an exceptional – although not unsurprising – low. Consumers want and deserve a more open system, in which they are active participants, rather than the current system of vested interests and party politics. Rational, informed public debate is not something that should be feared by Government; it is a pity that currently it is. In addition, the costs involved in setting up the agency would be saved by redirecting money from other government bodies – not that the BSE crisis was not very expensive itself.

A Wider Malaise?

But is this enough? Lead was not phased out of British petrol until effects of brain damage were found in British children – as if American evidence proving the same link did not apply on this side of the Atlantic. Given the long saga of misleading reassurance on BSE and similar issues – including phthalates in baby milk, faulty HIV tests, and the oral contraceptives disaster – that is scarcely surprising. It is not just health issues that the Government seems to mismanage – from asbestos to lead in petrol, from radiation to acid rain, from pesticides to threats to the ozone layer, even the arms to Iraq scandal – the Government's handling of matters stem from the culture of denial that is all too prevalent throughout the British establishment.

No-one claims that Britain is a dictatorship, or that it is fundamentally not a democracy, but there is now growing support for the thesis that the British constitution is outmoded for the twentieth century – let alone the twenty-first. At one time Britain was held as a shining model of democratic Government in action, and the US tri-polar system was based on our Monarch (President), Lords (Senate), and Commons (House of Representatives). In the past 200 years the rest of the developed world has adapted and changed with the times, experimenting with new forms of contract between elected and electors, different ways of checking and balancing the institutions of Government, and responding to wider access to higher quality education and the onset of mass media by opening up information about government and the decisions that are taken on behalf of the people. Britain, which always prided itself on its evolving, "organic" constitution, has not kept pace with the changes happening in other countries and in other business and commercial sectors. The BSE crisis is but the latest example of why we must wake up to this reality.

We need a Freedom of Information Act, independent Food and Drugs Commission and possibly a separate Department of Consumer Protection.

These are probably the best ways to prevent disasters such as the BSE crisis from happening again. The damage done by the Government's handling of the BSE crisis can, unfortunately, never be undone. Our health has been compromised, farmers have been ruined, our relations with the European Union have been soured further, and the beef industry will take many years to recover. Perhaps ministers will learn from the BSE fiasco; but don't bet on it. Bet instead, as long as the *status quo* exists, on a similar culture of denial over the next big threat – whatever it may be.

A good recent model is provided by Sweden. In 1992 the Swedish Parliament set up a National Institute of Public Health, whose main task is to engage in health promotion and disease prevention in close collaboration with national and local authorities as well as popular movements. Also, their Socialstyrelsen acts as an advisory and supervisory agency for the Government in the fields of health and social services. This agency follows up central Government initiatives to check they tally with the original aims. The Swedes, at least, have recognized that openness and co-operation is far more likely to yield positive results than the "secret society" of the UK.

And why can the Government not learn from the Swedish experience that freedom of information, rather than a "need to know" culture, prevents sensationalist scare stories rather than creates them?

Part III

Understanding the Crisis

Chapter 11

Madness, Metaphors and Miscommunication: The Rhetorical Life of Mad Cow Disease

Joan Leach

Writing about an event that is ongoing challenges the most confident cultural observer; but writing about an event that has, and may well again, claimed lives challenges both one's confidence and one's ethics. The BSE (bovine spongiform encephalopathy) "crisis" in Britain is just such an event. Calling it an event may even sound odd to the reader's ears, but it is a first step back in a process of observing the events of our time from a more remote position. Calling the ongoing spectacle over BSE a "crisis", which is a more familiar way of talking about it, is itself taking a quite different position on BSE, invoking the language of "health scares" and a discourse of control and containment. Each type of discourse comes from a position of thinking and action about the BSE issue in Great Britain. This chapter is about just that: the myriad positions that are available to those who want to talk about the BSE event. Each of these positions, including the one in this chapter, however, is not neutral and carries with it certain cultural assumptions and structuring metaphors. Like the classical Greek figure Procrustes, each metaphor limits or extends the ways that certain evidence can fit into an argument.[1] This chapter will look at the way that Procrustean practices are at work in the rhetoric of the BSE event. Some metaphors extend evidence too far to cover areas where the evidence may, in actuality, be too short. Other metaphors lop off evidence that may be applicable because it does not fit the structure of the metaphor.

The goal of this type of analysis is not to be "scientific" in the traditional sense of exacting observation, testing hypotheses, and making predictions. Nor should this analysis leave the reader with the feeling that if only we could purge all language, especially scientific language, of its metaphorical resonances we would be left with a language that is "accurate" and shows the "real" relationship between BSE and CJD (Creutzfeldt–Jakob disease), between medical science and the culture it proposes to treat, or even between language and reality. This chapter is to show the slipperiness of language and to highlight the metaphors and narratives which are currently used in the popular media to represent BSE to the majority of the populace. We do, however, have the power both to reflect on, and to change the metaphors we use in certain contexts. And while language seems all the more slippery when dealing with issues of scientific and cultural import, this is an awesome power indeed.

Rhetoric of Science as Cultural Observation

In the past ten years, scholars and experts in rhetoric have turned their attention to issues in science and medicine.[2] Rhetorical studies have long concentrated on the ways in which language is used to persuade, to console, and even to structure public opinion and discourse on matters of political and civic interest.[3] Figures such as Plato and Aristotle, as well as others like Gorgias and Prodicus in even earlier classical times concerned themselves with persuasion in the law courts and in political assemblies.[4] They claimed to be able to both analyze and teach persuasion to students who wanted to excel and find notoriety in being able to make persuasive arguments in controversial or uncertain situations. Since classical times, this "art of rhetoric" has enjoyed academic popularity as well as academic disdain as a theoretical position from which to analyze the persuasive "rhetoric" of politicians, soothsayers, and other public figures (Meyer 1994). As science has become one of the most prevalent areas of knowledge in the late twentieth century, it has also become the most authoritative source to quote as evidence for persuasive arguments. Rhetoricians have noticed this and have sought to find out how science functions in a persuasive context. (For a series of essays about science in a persuasive mode see Gross 1990.)

From rhetorical interest in science has come several observations about how science persuades through the use of language in scientific papers, monographs, and specialist congresses. Additionally, much has been written about the additional persuasive force that science has when used as evidence in popular sources such as popular science books, magazines, television and radio programmes, and in science museums. (For an in-depth analysis see Nelkin 1995.) Central to these discussions of the persuasive use of science are the forms of narrative in which science is placed, the role and representation of scientific uncertainty, and the key role of metaphor in both formal and popular science writing. These three aspects are useful for a rhetorical analysis of the scientific language surrounding BSE as they help to point out the ways in which BSE has been treated in popular representations that are similar to other "crises" and ways in which the language surrounding BSE is particular to this event.

The Narrative Context

BSE did not emerge into a culture unfamiliar with medical and scientific controversy. In the past five years, Great Britain has suffered from food and health scares including listeria in eggs, salmonella in chickens, fears about the risk of thrombosis from the birth control pill, and worries about genetically altered tomatoes in supermarket tomato paste. Indeed, health worries about AIDS, the emergence of antibiotic resistant strains of tuberculosis, and ethical concerns about xenotransplantation have dominated popular coverage of science and health issues in the broadsheet press. But *how* have they dominated? While it is certainly easily seen that good journalists tell a good story, it is less commonly noticed that the properties of narratives about science have many of the same features as fairy tales, films, and novels. Indeed, Paul Feyerabend (1978) noticed that even in the driest of scientific papers "style, elegance of expression, simplicity of presentation, tension of plot and narratives, and seductiveness of content become important features of our knowledge." How then, has the public become interested in BSE from the scientific data that has been collected and what are the "seductive" features drawing readers into the media narrative of BSE?

Who is the Author of BSE Narratives?

The structure of narrative is such that one of its first features noticed in a story is the narrative voice, that is, who it is that seems to be speaking through the text. Scientific papers have long been subjected to bemused scrutiny from colleagues in other disciplines for the strange conventions that they observe in relation to narrative voice: the use of the passive voice, no first person observations, strange jargon, the lack of connection with other events in the public sphere. In technical writing, the goal is to erase the author and remove the personal dimensions that authorship represents. When the author sneaks back in, she is greeted with scepticism. In the words of Scott Montgomery (1996b),

> Any point at which there emerges something resembling a truly personal or literary style in a technical article is commonly considered to be a point of failure, when required standards are transgressed and "scientific" discourse begins to break down. Among the scientific community, the personal excites a degree of suspicion, even discomfort or disdain.

This observation about the narrative voice is crucial to a rhetorical analysis of BSE. Who is it that is speaking and to whom at certain points during the "crisis" and how are they viewed by both a popular and media audience? There have been many "voices" who have been heard during this event, but here, we will focus on one individual who highlights the tension between authority and authorship, credibility, and disdain – Dr Harash Narang.

As the story of the connection between BSE and CJD became a popular media subject, the search for a scientist who would openly speak to the press was on. Such a figure presented himself in the person of Dr Harash Narang. Since late 1995, Dr Narang has been the object of both media adoration and abuse. No matter how one personally feels about the claims and the evidence proposed by Dr Narang, one has to admit that he has become one of the few recognizable scientific figures throughout the BSE debate. Dr Narang first made national British news when he claimed to have invented the first test for BSE in cattle in 1990. He claimed that "at this stage I found this quick diagnostic method. You would touch the surface of the brain and examine it in the electron microscope." This he called the "touch impression technique." From there, Narang was the subject of a *Close Up North* program on BBC TV. In 1995 he was guest expert on a *World in Action* documentary. He has been quoted in the *British Parliamentary Review*, has successfully enlisted the support of six Labour MPs and had the shadow agriculture minister actively campaigning on his behalf. He has recently become popular for another kind of test, a simple urine test, which he is urging to be used on cattle across the country to test for BSE. While he has been the spotlight of media attention and used as an expert by government ministers and the parents of ailing children with CJD, Narang has also been exposed as a purported "quack" by several science correspondents for British national daily newspapers. In mid-August 1996 Emily Green resigned from the *Independent* and wrote a feature expose for the *Guardian* entitled "A cow and bull story?" where she systematically discredited Narang and his purported science, critiquing her media colleagues for giving him national exposure and the position of an expert. To some, Narang is an harassed figure who has bravely fought the scientific elite claiming "right from the start of this crisis, the government has not approached BSE as a matter of science but as a matter of policy, viewing research as some kind of convenience store where you can pick and choose the hypotheses that suit you." To others, Harash Narang is a scientific impostor, schooled neither in the treatments of medical science nor the exactitudes of clinical epidemiology. His detractors would point out that he has cleverly claimed others' research as his own and has masqueraded these techniques as proven diagnostics for both BSE and CJD where either no proof is available, or, where proof is available, the techniques are redundant to clear symptoms of disease.

Such contested figures are not interesting for the potential benefits that they bring in terms of diagnostic or clinical success, as frequently they bring none. Indeed, some, like Emily Green, would go so far as to claim that any attention that they get is at the hands of inexperienced or unknowledgeable sources such as parliamentary ministers or journalists. But the figure of Harash Narang, from a narrative point of view, makes us pause. He is not alone among shadowy figures that appear in conflict or uncertain situations. Indeed, one thinks of Peter Duesberg in the AIDS crisis and numerous others of the cancer wars fame (see also Proctor 1996). One aspect highlighted by the tension between Narang's popular success and critical failure is the issue that he has violated the rules of scientific discourse and the conventions of scientific decorum with the press. As Montgomery alludes, Harang's patina of scientific credibility breaks down *because* he becomes a public figure. As such, he is subject to scientific incredulity and met with significant scepticism by the scientific establishment. As these norms become increasingly explicit, Narang begins to look suspect because he is "too" public; he is seen too often in front of a camera and not in a laboratory. He is talking of certainty while the remainder of the scientific community is speaking in terms of uncertainty. We will return to this notion of certainty and uncertainty in "crisis" situations and see the ways in which the "crisis" over BSE has turned the public's notion of certainty on its head.

As public figures, "rogue scientists" are inviting to the media and their readership for cultural and metaphorical reasons. As a scientific figure, Narang is the prototypical anti-hero, despised by the establishment, coming forward with bold theories and wild conjectures, campaigning on behalf of innocent victims, himself the victim of government conspiracy. Indeed, Harash Narang is the anti-hero of fairy tales.[5] Both media discourse and public discourse have adopted this narrative in talking about him. In the 2 March 1996 issue of *The Times*, Narang received press coverage of his demand to use his urine test on ailing patients to determine whether they have contracted CJD. The press reported in the same article that the rogue Narang had established a CJD campaign group with the families of victims Peter Hall, Morris Callaghan, Stephen Churgill, and Fonnie Van Es. The upshot was that Narang and his group of victims was ready to take matters into their own hands as the establishment was afraid to act. This was echoed in the letters section of that same newspaper when a member of the public wrote to insist that "if they simply used Harash Narang's methods there may well be a way of eliminating infected herds and not have a mass slaughter."

In addition to his anti-heroic status, he is needed as an expert for institutional reasons having to do with the structure of the press. Further, he is needed as an expert in a context where the role of the expert is undefined and in some cases, undisclosed. Who is the expert in the BSE/CJD arena of scientific expertise? Is it the epidemiologist, the molecular biologist, the veterinarian? Tom Wilkie, formerly of the *Independent*, now Senior Policy Analyst at PRISM (Centre for Policy Research in Science and Medicine), has indicated that during the early days of the BSE event, when SEAC (Spongiform Encephalopathy Advisory Committee) was first convened for a cloistered weekend to discuss the evidence before them and make policy decisions on the future of British beef, they effectively left no-one with secured "expert" status for the press to question for several days (Wilkie 1996). The press, therefore, turned to other "experts" including Dr Narang. The question of expertise and authority is a problematic one when dealing with questions of uncertainty. Science itself is supposed to offer certainty in the textual structure of its arguments. For example, as Jeanne Fahnestock (1986) has clearly shown, textual certainty in popular or "accommodated" accounts of certainty is produced in a double move. First, scientists are aware of multiple interpretations based on alternative readings of their data; they tend to show that they are aware of possible criticism and refutations that an expert audience could raise against their interpretation. To protect themselves from this refutation, the scientist usually authors sentences which acknowledge uncertainty including words such as "appears" or "suggests". Secondly, journalists have no pressure to respond or be aware of multiple interpretations of the same scientific findings. These "hedge" words tend to fall out in journalistic accounts, rendering the description of the scientific data more certain than it would otherwise have been. The scientist, therefore, is supposed to be an expert who can adjudicate between interpretative accounts and argue for one interpretation. The journalist, however, takes the argument at face value and elevates it to a kind of truth. This does not mean that journalists are necessarily "wrong" or that scientific expertise is misleading. However, it does mean that the scientific expert is placed in the role of judge and jury of alternative accounts of data. This kind of expertise, then, is especially powerful when used in popular reports of science where alternative accounts are effectively silenced by the lack of availability of alternative experts.

But the BSE story, like all good detective stories, adds a narrative twist to the scientific sleuthing for certainty. Being uncertain has gradually become the mark of the respected scientist while being certain is clear to brand one, as Harash Narang has found out the hard way, a quack or snake-oil salesman. From the quest for authority to the uneasy acceptance of uncertainty, the story of BSE has done much to revise the issue of uncertainty before a lay audience at a not previously acknowledged level of complexity and with a multiplicity of representations. Much as Collins & Pinch (1993) have pointed out in their sociological analyses of science, science – including medical science – "progresses" in fits and starts; but it needs to have a motivation to progress at all. In scientific medicine, that motivation is perhaps two-fold, first to find a cure, treatment, or prevention, and secondly, to have reasonable certainty about the efficacy of that cure, treatment, or prevention.[6] The narrative story of BSE has evolved from the beginning of the popular coverage of the crisis where a cure was demanded and certainty about the safety of British beef was desired. It became clear that neither cure nor certainty was immediately possible and that the scientific leaning toward uncertainty was the "reasonable" line to take. This is most clear from the first stories in the popular accounts of BSE to reach the public. In 1990, the editors of *Nature* chastised the Government saying, "Never say there is no risk. Instead, say that there is always risk. The problem really is to calculate what it is. Never say that the risk is negligible unless you are sure that your listeners share your own philosophy of life." The editors clearly felt that the Government had expressed certainty when the evidence demanded a more uncertain line. Since then, the Government has taken to talking about "safety" and not certainty. MAFF (Ministry of Agriculture, Fisheries and Food) quotes John Pattison, the chairman of SEAC as saying "In any common usage of the word, beef is safe." The focus is not on risk because popular representations have concentrated on risk and have rather effectively showed that current scientific knowledge could not eliminate "risk". However, "safety" is another matter altogether. The narrative features of the narrative voice, here the scientific authority or expert, and the subtext of uncertainty provide a rhetorical context for the BSE "event". However, we must also look to the structure of the story, the narrative features of BSE itself.

We have a Suspect Hero, What is the Story-line?

The "facts" of BSE can be described in the following scientific and medical terminology: fatal, long incubation period, degenerative pathology, no antibody response, unconventional agents, afebrile, lesions in the CNS (central nervous system), no inflammatory response.[7] However, these "facts" do not make sense in and of themselves. They need to be woven into some kind of "story" or narrative which makes sense of them in the context of other "facts" and social contexts. Indeed, as a popular narrative the BSE story-line has much in common with other disease narratives such as AIDS, the recent re-emergence of tuberculosis, cancer, and other devastating illnesses. That their narratives seem similar may have something to do with the "facts" of the disease; but again, the metaphors we use tend to structure our narratives to look similar.

Key Metaphors Structuring BSE Representations

Popular representations of science have always been rife with metaphors, similes, analogies, and explanations in familiar terms drawn from the world of experience, some of which have been less than edifying, as Scott Montgomery (1996a) indicates:

> as carnival facts ("As many as 230 million such bacteria would fit on a single pencil dot"); the most banal familiarities, for example, those of the kitchen ("Once the batter of the earth congealed"), the TV drama or soap opera ("Particle interactions can be seen as a series of marriages and divorces"), or the neighbourhood ("In the second decade of this century, we learned that our sun resides in the suburbs of a galaxy"); storybook imagery ("At that time, huge carnivorous monsters filled the seas"), military simile ("Our bodies are under constant attack from unseen chemicals"), or, of course, the sports science ("Once the catalytic whistle goes off, various molecular teams go into motion").

These metaphors are not always as banal as those witnessed above. Susan Sontag (1977) has pointed out the dangerous, misleading, and culturally significant metaphors associated with cancer. Similarly, Paula Treichler (1989) has examined the metaphorical resonances of AIDS as an "epidemic of signification". Again, powerful war imagery, homophobic language, and an overwhelming sense of frustration and impotence in the face of disease is conveyed through the predominating metaphors.[8] So, while frequently it is tempting to talk of metaphors as consciously invoked figures that popular writers and journalists use to simplify and make familiar complex and foreign topics, Sontag (1977) and Triechler (1989), as well as others, have given examples of the structuring and constitutional function of metaphors and figurative language. Two such structuring metaphors in the BSE popular media coverage is madness and the metaphorical relationship between humans and animals.

Metaphorically Mad

In what sense can "madness" be a metaphor? A metaphor is most commonly a figure of speech by which a word or phrase is applied to an object or action that it does not literally denote in order to imply that in fact, a resemblance exists. It operates in some cases like a transference of a set of characteristics from one thing to another thing with different characteristics. In English, "mad" usually has two dominant meanings, one approximating being angry, and the other approximating crazy. The latter is much more common in British English than in American English. Madness also includes a particular fondness as in "I'm mad about you" or can even apply to an animal with rabies as in "mad dogs". In literature and popular representations of madness, the afflicted tear their hair, act foolishly, destructively, or in such a way to cause harm to themselves or others. In other words, the "mad" act outside the conventions of normal behavior. This is the denotative use of the word "mad" and its possible applications. The richness of the word "mad", however, comes from a rich connotative history where scientists are "mad", "Ophelia" was "mad", and women can be "mad". That is, "madness" is not just acting outside the norms or conventions of behavior, it is a normative statement that can be made against someone or something. This image of the "mad scientist" for example, does not simply evoke the image of a crazy or mentally deranged person. It conjures the image of a brilliant genius who will use that genius for depraved or unsavoury purposes. In this way, "madness" picks up metaphorical connotations that come along with the application of the word "mad" in other situations. In one sense, cows who have been affected with BSE do act outside the normal conventions of cow behavior. They are mad in this narrow sense. But the context of the application of the word "mad" changes its meaning. We usually do not refer to cows as "mad" even when they do behave outside cow-like conventions. Why is this important for the media representations of BSE? For one, the word "mad" has applied to humans, cows, minks, scientists, and politicians throughout the BSE media event and with relative indiscrimination. There is a sense in which the BSE event becomes a "crisis" because everything is "mad". That is, all systems are operating out of the ordinary conventions; thus, the title appearing in the *Observer on Sunday*, "It's a Mad, Mad, Mad, Maff world" and the more figurative *Guardian* title "Mad Cows & Englishmen" (*Guardian* 8 December 1995).

In addition to this meaning of "madness" as out of the ordinary or unconventional, however, is the strange sense in which cows can be "mad" at all. Other than the use of the word "mad" to describe animals with rabies, "madness" is a human attribute. Mad cow disease is thus an anthropomorphism of sorts, making the connection between cows and humans. The following example from the *Guardian* (8 December 1995) highlights the way in which referring to cows as "mad" heightens the sense of human danger,

> People who ate infected meat in the late 1980's may not show signs of the disease until the next millennium. Then, if the doomsday scenarios proved right, biblical numbers could suffer loss of co-ordination, intellect and personality – just like the wobbly mad cows seen on TV.

The "madness" in this paragraph clearly describes the behavior of humans, not those of the cows. The cows on TV were wobbly, but in what sense did they suffer a loss of intellect or personality? These are typically human attributes and giving them to cows heightens the sense of loss to humans. It is as if the term "mad cow" was originally coined to demonstrate the loss of cognitive capacity to the cows, to resonate with the sense of madness in animals as in rabies, and to be a humorous "hook" for newspaper stories. Now that the question of the transmission of BSE from cows to humans has been broached, however, the connotations are no longer humorous, but horrific, "Victims of the human equivalent of 'mad cow' disease face a horrific death – they go slowly mad and they die as their brains are riddled with holes" (Reuters 27 March 1996). We rhetorically gave a human attribute to an animal and now it comes back to suggest our own fate in a manner more horrific than if we had perhaps described it another way.

Human and Animal

To elaborate even more on this metaphorical transference of characteristics, let us look more closely at the issue of transmission. Among popular representations of BSE, the image of the cow stumbling through the mud, unable to stand, and swaying to and fro has become a powerful image and metaphor for the possibility for human disease in the form of CJD. The analogy clearly goes, like cow, like human. As the BSE event has "progressed", increased concern was voiced about the transmissiveness of BSE to humans in the form of CJD. The technical mode and method of such transmission is still hotly debated and the frequency of possible transmission actively contested. However, the image of the staggering cow has been coupled with the image of dying CJD victims in hospitals with considerable frequency in both video and print media. It has also done much to both blur the distinction between "animal" and human diseases as well as heighten awareness of a range of issues that are currently being debated in the British media on the issues of human and animal nature.

Here, BSE connects to media interest in other areas involving animals and humans. Most notably, transgenic organ transplant between animals and humans which was famously symbolized by the "ear-mouse" picture which ran on the front page of nearly every British daily newspaper. The Nuffield report on the ethics of xenotransplantation even made the connection between xenotransplantation and BSE alluding to BSE's ability to jump the species barrier (Nuffield Council on Bioethics Report 1996). If it can happen with BSE and we are introducing animal parts into humans, might we not run the risk of spreading diseases across species, the argument went. These are not inconsequential comparisons as human treatment of animals is central to this metaphorical dyad – like animals, like humans.

One of the arguments structured by this metaphor is the argument about the ethical treatment of animals and the agricultural practices that have been spotlighted as a potential cause of BSE as well as its persistence. Advocates have claimed that BSE is the punishment reaped for many years of poor agricultural practice. More radical arguments have included that this is the wrath of nature for eating beef at all; a *Sunday Times* article ran under the title "Nature's Revenge" and started with the leader, "Nature has a habit of inflicting retribution on those who break its rules" (17 December 1995). Clearly, not only the health of the populace is at stake, but also the boundaries between animal and human, *Homo* and bovine. Mary Douglas (1975) has argued that the typical human reaction to disorder which includes reactions to risk, contradictions, and uncertainties is classification. By creating categories to explain the disorder, the system can be repaired; order is restored. Perhaps this is what we are seeing in the rhetoric of the BSE event. In response to uncertainty introduced by the possibility of disease passed between species, one rhetorical strategy is to renegotiate the boundaries between species and negotiate the proper treatment each species should receive.

Narrative Closure

Heightening the uncertainty felt by the public about the BSE event, the media and science have not yet ended the story. The BSE event offers no narrative closure, no ending by which the truth is recovered, boundaries stabilized, or uncertainty made certain. This should make us ever more watchful about the metaphors and narratives of BSE. It is, as Nietzsche said, "the metaphors of the past that become the truth of the present." In medical science, in science, and in the press, it is the power of metaphor which constructs and constrains the possible stories which we tell. Metaphorical power creates lasting images and entire systems of images. The cow stumbling through the mud coupled with the 18-year-old boy in his hospital bed is central to our understanding of BSE as well as a symbol in which we negotiate our relationship with animals and how we treat them. It does not mean that metaphors are all we have or that through metaphorical understanding we will have an answer to the problem of BSE. But it is by considering how the stories, terms, and images that have arisen in relation to BSE that will enable us to see how non-technical issues organize and constrain the patterns of our thought and the potentialities of our solutions, to have our revenge on Procrustean metaphors.

Notes

1 Procrustes was a legendary figure from Greek antiquity who was said to have lived on the road between Athens and Eleusis. He seduced strangers with the kindest of hospitality then seized them and fastened them to a bed. He made them fit the bed, if it was not to their size, by cutting short their limbs if they were too long for it, or putting them on a rack to stretch if they were too short.

2 Issues of rhetorical interest in Health Communication have been flagged by Judith Segal in "Patient Compliance, the Rhetoric of Rhetoric, and the Rhetoric of Persuasion" in *Rhetoric Society Quarterly* Summer/Fall 1993: 90–102 and Kathryn Montgomery Hunter in *Doctor's Stories: The Narrative Structure of Medical Knowledge*. Princeton: Princeton University Press, 1991.

3 John Poulakos' *Sophistical Rhetoric in Classical Greece*, Columbia: University of South Carolina Press, 1995 is a good introduction to the origins of rhetoric as a classic analytic and political practice.

4 Indeed, the *agora*, or public square of Greek political life was not empty of scientists and physicians, either. The Hippocratic corpus, written from the 5th century to the 2nd century BC, is riddled with allusions to physicians who communicated for a living. There were two chief reasons for this: first, Greek medicine acknowledged that a healthy person was also a healthy citizen. To be a healthy citizen, one must make their voice heard in the *agora*. Thus, the ability for rhetoric, or communication, was a mark of health. Secondly, the ancient physician was judged by the public and his future patients in the *agora* where he was expected to debate with other physicians about particular techniques and healing cures to be used while practicing the art of medicine.

5 Dr Narang is not alone among researchers who have been given an heroic role in the BSE event. The 28 May 1994 issue of *New Scientist* blazes with the title fit for another potential anti-hero, Dr Stanley Prusiner: "Mad brains and the prion heresy: The idea that a simple protein could act as an infectious agent was too much for most biochemists. Georgina Ferry reports on what happened when one man dared to go out on a limb." Other unlikely heros include Richard Lacey who has had a similar trajectory as Harash Narang.

6 Collins & Pinch (1993) describe science as a Golem. The Golem is a creature from Jewish mythology who goes forward in the world in a haphazard manner. The Golem is neither evil nor good, but may be either given the context in which it is placed. What motivates it on is a word scratched into its

forehead, TRUTH. The parallel here is with certainty. While certainty is the goal for science, it is not always clear how that certainty will be achieved and to what ultimate end, good or evil.

7 Indeed, these were the terms that were highlighted by Professor Douglas Young in his lecture to the British Association for the Advancement of Science Annual Meeting, Birmingham, 12 September 1996.

8 However, popular representations are not alone in using cultural stereotypes as bases for scientific analogy and metaphor. Biology and medicine have been heavily scrutinized for the powerful gendered metaphors that they use. See Bonnie Spanier, *Im/Partial Science* (Bloomington: Indiana University Press, 1996) for a careful analysis of gendered metaphors in molecular biology.

References

Collins, H. & T. Pinch 1993. *The Golem: what everyone should know about science*. Cambridge: Cambridge University Press.

Douglas, M. 1975. *Implicit meanings: essays in anthropology*. London: Routledge.

Fahnestock, J. 1986. Accommodating science. *Written Communication* (July), 275–96.

Feyerabend, P. 1978. *Against method*. London: Verso.

Gross, A. 1990. *The rhetoric of science*. London: Harvard University Press.

Meyer, M. 1994. *Rhetoric, language and reason*. University Park: Pennsylvania State University Press.

Montgomery, S. L. 1996. The cult of jargon: reflections on language in science. In *The scientific voice*, S.L. Montgomery (ed.), 1–69. London: Guildford Press.

Nelkin, D. 1995. *Selling science*. London: Freeman.

Nuffield Council on Bioethics Report 1996. *Animal to human transplants: the ethics of xenotransplantation*. London.

Proctor, R. L. 1996. *Politics and the cancer wars*. New York: Basic Books.

Sontag, S. 1977. *Illness as metaphor*. London: Penguin.

Triechler, P. 1989. AIDS: an epidemic of signification. In *AIDS, Homophobia and Biomedical Discourse*. Boston: MIT.

Wilkie, T. 1996. *How the media covered BSE*. British Association for the Advancement of Science Annual Meeting, Birmingham, 12 September 1996.

Chapter 12, part i

Media Coverage of the Mad Cow Issue: Introduction

J. Gregory Payne

There is no doubt that the scare was hyped up. Certainly that would be the instinct of most journalists to hype the story rather than play a socially responsible role in relating the issue. (George Parker, journalist *The Financial Times*)[1]

The power of the media in influencing or, as some would vociferously argue, in determining our reality, is a subject of interest that has generated both serious scholarly academic inquiry and popular debate and discussion. Few would contest the premise that today's journalists have an awesome responsibility, given their two-fold and sometimes competitive function of informing the public and being the first to do so in an era of instantaneous global communication.

The mad cow crisis provides an intriguing context and case study for those interested in the agenda-setting phenomenon and its impact on a global public policy issue. In addition, it is an opportunity to examine the print media's performance in providing meaning to a fast-breaking story with global consequences. What types of claims were made in the announcement stage of this story? What evidence was offered to support the claims that, pieced together, provided meaning for a public anxious to know and emerged as the mosaic of meaning in understanding the facts surrounding the mad cow issue?

Was there a difference in the print media product in Britain from that offered readers in the United States? If so, is it a reflection of cultural differences? Does proximity to the crisis affect the reporting style and performance? What did the US national press report? Were there distinctions in coverage between Britain and the US, in general, and regionally within America among its papers? Were there differences in tone of the news coverage, i.e. objective, straightforward reporting of the facts; or editorialized criticism offered by the reporter in a given newspaper?

It is these and other relevant questions that the media analysis that follows by Veronica Demko and Daniel Dornbusch attempts to examine. In highlighting such coverage in the UK, Mr Dornbusch examines the emergence of the BSE issue and its coverage in one of Britain's most factual publications, the *Financial Times*. Mr Dornbusch selected this publication due to its international readership and *The Times* tendency to downplay the British tabloid journalistic style of incorporating political viewpoints within news coverage. Ms Demko's study focuses on a content analysis of five major US newspapers: *The New York Times, Chicago Tribune, Los Angeles Times, The Wall Street Journal* and the *Washington Post*.

Previous Research

The influence of media coverage on a public's understanding and the emerging meaning of a public policy issue is supported in past academic research. A domestic study examining the media coverage of an American public policy pronouncement on Medicare concluded, "Such questions are pertinent and warrant investigation given the fact that the popular press, in their role as artists of the mediated reality, chiefly provide the meaning of such matters of policy making to the general public" (Payne et al. 1989). Offering further insight on the relationship of press coverage and public awareness, McCombs notes that "If the media tell us nothing about a topic or event, then in most cases it simply will not exist on our personal agenda or in our life space" (McCombs & Shaw 1976). Furthermore, Susan Herbst (1997) in her forthcoming book on the role of the media in policy making and public opinion writes, "The social climate, technological milieu, and communication environment in any democratic state together determine the way we think about public opinion and the ways we try to measure it."

Support for these viewpoints reach into the market place of policy making. Linsky (1986) found that of more than 500 former government officials and policy-makers interviewed, 96% identified the press as having a substantial impact on federal policy. More importantly, he noted a relationship between the type of press coverage and its impact on policy making: favorable news stories facilitated an idea being transformed into actual policy while negative news stories prolonged the decision-making process. Given the recognized role of journalists in influencing not only public opinion but the policy-making process, examination of the coverage of the mad cow crisis can provide insight for those interested in political communication.

In the media analyses to follow, a chronological trend summary can shed light on the emerging public meaning and understanding of the BSE incident. The announcement and definition phase characterize the first mention of the news event and the characteristics associated with it. Of particular interest to those examining the emergence of meaning and understanding are the arguments – claims, warrants and evidence or data – offered to the public in this initial coverage. It is important to examine the causal links implied as well as stated in such arguments in the effort to fully appreciate their continued presence, modification, or rejection as the story further develops with additional

information, verification by lay and scientific measures of questionable assertions, and changing environmental contexts. The product of such deliberation is
"meaning" for the public.

It is within this definition phase that generalizations and value judgments
are offered concerning agents involved in the newsworthy event. In addition,
one learns the degree of co-ordination, if any, of the various persuasive
strategies by the responsible agents/agencies connected with the story in
addressing issues raised in the announcement phase. Is there a recognition of
the power of the media in helping get the message out to the public by those
agents and agencies responsible for the announcement? How well is the press
coverage product – the mediated image – controlled by the agent/agency? What
is the evaluation of such agents by the press in the coverage offered?

"Debunking" follows the announcement and definition phases. This
critical stage is characterized by careful scrutiny of any uncertain aspect of, or
claim within, a story. Sometimes a noted change in tone occurs precipitated by
the press taking on a more adversarial relationship in its attempt to provide the
public the "facts" needed for deliberative decision making. In many instances
of debunking, controversial claims or assertions are merely dropped in coverage
owing to the lack of supportive evidence or the "conventional wisdom" that
such an interpretation should no longer be offered.

Trends in the Coverage

The *Financial Times*

Examination of the *Financial Times* coverage reveals the announcement and
definition phase of coverage focused – in editorials and in news stories – on the
lack of governmental co-ordination in explaining the governmental plan and the
economic impact of the crisis. In what appears to be a knee-jerk response to a
story appearing in the tabloid style *Daily Mirror*, which announced the link of
BSE (bovine spongiform encephalopathy) or mad cow disease to CJD
(Creutzfeldt-Jakob disease), the British Ministry of Health scheduled an ill-
advised and ill-planned news conference. The ensuing messages – (1) that
British beef was safe, (2) but that millions of cattle would be destroyed –
invited speculation and comment from the press, lay people and the scientific
community. The result was a scientific link – real or imagined – between BSE
and CJD in the ensuing coverage. This was established as a major focus of the
coverage during the first month within the announcement and definition phases.
The mediated image of BSE was similar to the threat and deaths associated with
the AIDS epidemic, a theme which permeated news stories and editorials during
the initial weeks of coverage.

A leading scientist predicted over one million deaths due to the crisis. Even
in the staid *Financial Times,* the impact of BSE was compared to the radioactive
fallout generated by the accident at Chernobyl. In the first month – the

announcement and definition phases – the link between BSE and CJD was the most prevalent theme in the examined coverage. Only in the debunking phase – which occurred months following the initial announcement – did the inferential link between BSE and CJD become weaker owing to a lack of verifiable scientific proof and skepticism by the media.

In the mad cow case, the Government in general and the British Ministry of Health in particular experienced a credibility gap with long-term ramifications. As an authoritative source, its nebulous message created doubt among journalists, the British public, domestic politicians and diverse publics within the European Union.

One lesson learned in this case is that it is mandatory to provide verified and factual information from a credible source to support emotional and controversial claims during the announcement/definition stage of the media coverage. Without faith in the source of the message – the British Ministry of Health – or guidance from credible experts, the media tended to seek out explanations which often were based more on speculation than hard science. The result, according to Mr Dornbusch, was that "British newspapers misrepresented the health risks." This misrepresented claim would also be a dominant characteristic of coverage found in the US. Integral to this issue was the proclivity of copy editors to further exaggerate the health risk in banner headlines that caught the eye of the public, albeit with a questionable claim in terms of accuracy or reliability. As Dornbusch illustrates, such inaccuracies in the British press reports heightened public fear in the earlier days of the crisis.

From an organizational perspective, Mr Dornbusch's analysis highlights the failure of the British Ministry of Health and the Ministry of Agriculture, Fisheries and Food to develop an appropriate media plan for the domestic and European public. The message of the press conference lacked clarity and credibility. It invited the press to "fill in the blanks" in the coverage and meaning it offered to the public.

In addition, the mistake of not notifying the appropriate members of the European Community concerning the BSE issue prior to the press conference proved to have tragic long term ramifications for British–European Union (EU) relations which were already strained prior to this announcement. The result of the specious claims presented in the press conference was an alarmed public that relied more on the press than the Government to supply information and prescriptions for containment of the crisis. In effect, the British media, rather than the British Government, became the primary source of information providing the public with meaning to the crisis in its reporting. The Government's inability to control the agenda, or even to influence it to any credible degree in weaving the web of meaning to the public, placed it in a reactive mode from the beginning and from which it has never recovered.

The governmental incompetence theme proved to be a major focus within much of the press coverage. This theme permeated editorials during the first announcement and definition phases of the crisis. The governmental agency's lack of credibility – or ethos as Aristotle labeled it over two thousand years ago

– compounded the problem which was to have damaging effects on the Conservative party as well as the political career of Prime Minister John Major.

US Newspaper Coverage

Ms Demko's study of the BSE coverage of five major US newspapers highlights what the author identifies as the "opposing pressures" facing journalists. Specifically, according to Demko, the "mad cow" issue presents journalists with a complicated news story devoid of any "hard" evidence that linked the major claims with the presented data. The story unfolded in the US within a context of growing governmental skepticism, in general, and a public's penchant for concise news nuggets that, at times, simplified rather than adequately explained the breaking newsworthy issues. Ms Demko identifies a general trend in American coverage to focus on a particular theme – of this as a story with distinct British identity, rather than the potential threat of the mad cow issue to the US public. Furthermore, the American press frequently used common images or topoi previously introduced by British journalists in detailing the chronology of the mad cow incident to readers.

Demko identifies a major characteristic of American coverage to be summed up as follows: the mad cow crisis is not of concern to Americans. Simply stated, BSE was a British problem, reflective of the British culture and general history of the British people; it was a product of what some reporters would claim was an "overindulgence of beef". In headlines, story themes and context, American coverage furthered the mediated image that the BSE–CJD controversy was deeply rooted in British norms and mores. As Demko illustrates with various metaphors, headlines and story themes, the result of such coverage was to communicate to American readers that BSE–CJD was a "British problem". It is not one of concern to Americans whose beef consumption is "not excessive", as is the present and historical case of our British cousins. In addition, the mad cow story and its context prodded some American journalists to advocate alternative eating habits in the American coverage of BSE.

Overall, the American press, as reflected in Demko's study, perpetuated the link between BSE and CJD in its general coverage but not to the extent of the British coverage. Even though the *New York Times* and *Washington Post* frequently provided qualifiers such as "might be linked" and "likely", the synoptic coverage offered by the American newspapers echoed that of the British counterparts. The coverage, Demko concluded, "turned what had been viewed as a veterinary problem into a potentially human one." It should be pointed out that none of the eight stories constituting the *Wall Street Journal* coverage – the least of any American newspaper examined – included a reference to particular cases of CJD associated with BSE.

Evidence for this BSE–CJD association in American coverage was familiar to that found in the British press. American coverage focused on the infamous 20 March 1996 announcement by British Health Ministry as the beginning point of the story. In US coverage, as in that of British stories, this was the defining moment in establishing the unsubstantiated link between BSE and CJD. Few if any US stories focused on the lack of scientific data, the uncertainty, or the contextual backdrop that characterized the initial announcement.

Keeping it simple for the American readers, US coverage identified the cause of the mad cow crisis as a product of governmental inefficiency: (1) in not forbidding the use of contaminated feed by its farmers, and (2) in the Government's inept manner as reflected in the March press conference.

Regarding the amount of coverage, Demko found the *New York Times* to reflect its international and paper of record reputation. Nearly four times as many articles (80) appeared in the *New York Times* as did in those papers which carried the next largest number of mad cow related stories – the *Chicago Tribune* and the *Los Angeles Times*.

This overview highlights the disturbing trend found in the mad cow coverage of both the British and US papers to perpetuate the questionable claim of the 1996 press conference establishing a link between BSE and CJD. While reflecting distinctive journalistic and cultural perspectives, such coverage not only set the agenda of the press, but also had a profound affect on policy making and politics in Britain and within the EU. Such analyses illustrate the importance of governmental agencies in assessing rhetorical strategies, co-ordinating such efforts, and providing credible suport for any controversial claims with potentially damaging impact. These steps were ignored by the British Government in March 1996.

The rhetorical residue of such inaction is evident. Almost one year after the British Ministry's press conference, a *New York Times* story, headlined, "British Government Faces New Accusation on Mad Cow Disease", wrote of the "collapse of confidence in the quality of a product (beef) for which Britain was long famous." Citing the criticism of the European Commision for the way in which the government had handled the situation, writer Warren Hodge, centered on the widening exigence of credibility or ethos initiated by the mad cow incident:

> When will someone in this Government take responsibility for the proper and competent administration of our affairs?

Notes

1 Interview with George Parker of the *Financial Times*. 28 January 1997.

References

Herbst, S. 1997. Theories of public opinion. Lecture given at the Joan Shorenstein Center on the Press, *Politics and Public Policy*, 10 March.

Linsky, M. 1986. *Impact: How the press affects federal policymaking.* New York: W.W. Morton.

McCombs, M.E. & D.L. Shaw 1976. Structuring the unseen environment. *Journal of Communication* **26**, 18–22.

Payne, J.G., S.C. Ratzan & R.A. Baukus, 1989. Dissemination of News in the Harvard Medicare Project: Regional/Discreet Differences. *Health Communication* **1**,(4).

An Analysis of Media Coverage of the BSE Crisis in Britain

Daniel Dornbusch

Summary Information from the British Ministry

Public awareness and perception of health risks depend upon the accuracy of health information reports, the reputation of the source, and the way the information is conveyed. This study of the *Financial Times'* coverage of the 1996 bovine spongiform encephalopathy (BSE) or "mad cow disease" indicates how inaccuracies in British press reports heightened public fear in the early days of the crisis. The public reaction, in turn, caused the government to respond with very severe measures to control the disease. The *Financial Times* stated that the consequences of "the crisis of Bovine Spongiform Encephalopathy, or mad cow disease, are more cataclysmic ... than the 1960s epidemic of foot-and-mouth disease, or the outbreak of salmonella and the Chernobyl radioactive fallout in the 1980s" (25 March, The culling of Britain's cattle).

The severe economic depression of Britain's cattle industry continues. The political ramifications stressed British international relations as "Euroskeptics" found increasing reason to voice criticisms. The Ministry of Agriculture lost considerable credibility with the public, in having to react to inaccurate news articles rather than taking the lead in providing accurate information, and possibly being able to apply more appropriate proactive measures, thereby decreasing the public fear and economic impacts. This study examines *Financial Times* coverage of BSE from January to September 1996.

Introduction and Sequence of Crucial Events

According to the *Financial Times* the British Ministry of Health continually assured the public that British beef posed absolutely no risk to humans from about 1988 until March 1996. The assurance was based on the available information at the time. However, there was some concern that BSE, or "mad cow disease" might actually pose a risk to human health.

In March 1996, the Spongiform Encephalopathy Advisory Committee (SEAC) together with representatives from the Creutzfeldt–Jakob disease (CJD)

Surveillance Unit, reported to the British Ministry of Health that BSE in fact was potentially dangerous to humans. Ten cases of a new variant of CJD, a spongiform encephalopathy, had been reported in Britain. The cause of this new disease was unknown. Without scientific evidence, SEAC proposed that the most likely cause of the new disease was BSE-ridden beef consumed before the 1989 restrictions imposed on cattle feed and slaughter.

The British public first learned of the SEAC report on 20 March 1996 when the *Daily Mirror* printed an article that effectively linked BSE with CJD. Later that day, the Ministry of Health held a press conference and made an official statement regarding SEAC's recommendations. Although the SEAC's report was received by the Government days before,[1] it was evident that the press conference was unscheduled. Twenty minutes before the conference, Mr Hogg, the British Agricultural minister, informed Mr Fischler, the European Union's Agricultural Commissioner, about the SEAC report and the ensuing statement. It became widely publicized that Mr Fischler was furious at Mr Hogg for not giving him ample time to analyze the data and prepare his own position. The Government's position was that British beef was safe to eat.[2] However, simultaneously, the Government mentioned that destroying a large portion of the British beef herd may be necessary.[3]

Some of the scientific community reported that the health risks of BSE were suspect. In a widely publicized television interview, Dr John Pattison, a leading scientist in encephalopathies, estimated that almost one half million people could die from the new CJD variant. The interviewer asked him if this "epidemic" could be as big as AIDS. Pattison said yes, but did not elaborate. With almost no evidence on the dangers of BSE or even the new variant of CJD, scientists and doctors were left guessing. Nevertheless, the public witnessed a leading scientist testify on national television that the CJD "epidemic" could be as deadly and widespread as AIDS.

Clearly, neither the scientific community nor the British Health Ministry disseminated accurate information about BSE quickly or effectively enough. In some instances the British press filled the information vacuum with misinformation about the dangers, heightening the public's fear. Indeed, it may be that the British media was partially responsible for creating the "mad-cow" crisis.

Did the British Media Shape BSE Perception?

The British media was analyzed for its creation or perpetuation of inaccurate BSE facts. Because of the sheer volume of BSE media reports, a single representative print medium was analyzed in this study. A broad examination of the many British news publications was considered neither possible nor necessary to obtain a reasonable understanding of the British press' affect on public opinion. Most carried similar accounts and one, the *Financial Times*, was chosen as it was considered to be among the most reliable.

British periodicals tend to incorporate political views into news reports much more prominently than others. To analyze the British media's conveyance of the BSE crisis accurately, it was imperative to find a periodical that minimized journalists' political views. A periodical with an extensive international readership was believed to represent a more balanced view of British politics. International readers would probably be more interested in British politics without biased political views. The *Financial Times* fits this profile with an estimated global readership of 1.3 million in 160 countries.[4]

The *Financial Times* has a firm tradition in unbiased reporting. Indeed within Britain the *Financial Times* has a strong reputation for seeking to provide unbiased reports. According to Julia Cuthbertson, news editor for the *Financial Times*, she seeks "What is the truth about any given set of information that we need to convey to our readers" (25 January 1997). Unlike "tabloid" periodicals, the *Financial Times* prides itself in producing analyses without exaggerating facts or omitting information to increase sales. It was therefore considered as a reasonable benchmark of ethical and responsible journalism.

The Nexis periodical database was screened for *Financial Times* articles on the BSE crisis spanning nine months, January through September 1996. Keywords "beef" and "mad cow" were used with the Boolian operator "or" to retrieve articles with either keyword. These terms were used because, together, they appeared to encompass every article that mentioned the BSE scare. Articles which briefly mentioned BSE were considered also because even a brief or humorous mention could convey false information to the reader, thus instilling inaccurate facts.

A total of 425 *Financial Times* articles were considered. The criteria used for analysis are generally referred to as: (a) type; (b) scientific link; (c) media image; (d) hysteria; (e) blame given; (f) Government competence. Each criteria is described in more detail in the Appendix.

Because judgments in determining to what degree these criteria were met are subjective, two different people analyzed the same information according to the criteria. Ratings were determined at a consistency level of 95%.

Results

A. Type of article

The results of analysis of the type of the article are shown in Tables 12.1 and 12.2. Table 12.1 shows the overall total number of articles of each type and the respective percentage of the total. Table 12.2 shows the breakdown of total articles by month. Particularly of note are the number of editorials published in each month: in March 17% of articles were editorials, in April 15%, whereas in May only 7% were editorials. There were nine articles that did not fit into the five categories. These were humorous anecdotes or quotations.

Table 12.1 Type overall totals

Type	Total number of articles	Percentage of total
News	256	60.2
Analysis	23	5.4
Editorial	54	12.7
Letter	12	2.8
Non-BSE	71	16.7
Other	9	2.2
Total	425	100.0

Table 12.2 Type totals by month, 1996

Type	Jan	Feb	March	April	May	June	July	August	Sept	Total
News	6	8	63	52	30	27	21	18	31	256
Analysis	0	0	5	4	4	4	1	3	2	23
Editorial	0	0	17	14	5	4	6	2	6	54
Letter	0	0	4	5	2	0	0	0	1	12
Non-BSE	0	1	11	20	26	2	0	1	10	71
Other	1	0	1	0	3	0	2	2	0	9
Total	7	9	101	95	70	37	30	26	50	425

B. Scientific link

The measurement of scientific linking between BSE and CJD are shown in Figure 12.1 and Table 12.3. Figure 12.1 indicates how the link was portrayed each month. Articles portraying a link are listed as a per cent per month.

Table 12.3 indicates the total number of articles by month that include mention of a "definite" link between diseases. All of these articles were published after the ministerial announcement on 20 March 1996.

Table 12.3 Number of articles by month mentioning a "definite" link, 1996

Month	Jan	Feb	March	April	May	June	July	August	Sept
No. of Articles	0	0	15	3	2	0	0	0	2

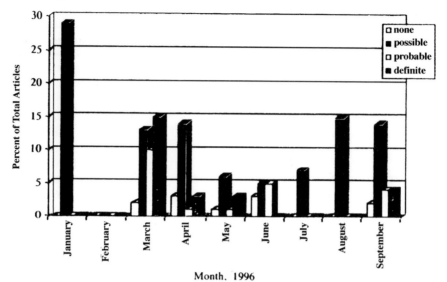

Figure 12.1 Mention of link between diseases, percent by month, 1996

Table 12.4 Subject totals

Media Subject	Total Number of Articles	Percent of Total
Scientific	22	5.2
Government wrangling	65	15.3
Euroskeptic	7	1.6
Plan of Government	147	34.6
Economic	124	29.2
Other	60	14.1
Total	425	100.0

C. Subject portrayed

Results of the analysis for the subject portrayed are shown in Tables 12.4 and 12.5. Table 12.4 illustrates the total number of articles of each image as well as the percentage of the total. Not every article contained a media subject. For example, not every article focused on economic factors or a plan of British Government. Media subject is further described in the Appendix. The articles without a media subject included most non-BSE-related articles and all humorous articles.

Table 12.5 shows the total number of articles by month of each category.

Table 12.5 Subject totals by month, 1996

Subject	Jan	Feb	March	April	May	June	July	August	Sept	Total
Science report	0	0	4	3	5	2	0	4	4	22
Govern. wrangling	0	0	16	16	6	9	5	3	10	65
Eurosk.	0	0	2	1	2	1	0	0	1	7
Plan of Govern.	0	4	20	37	23	18	17	7	21	147
Economy	6	5	53	25	11	4	7	5	8	124
Other	1	0	6	13	23	3	1	7	6	60
Total	7	9	101	95	70	37	30	26	50	425

D. Fear augmented

Results of analysis for the effect on public fear are shown in Table 12.6 and Figure 12.2. This table indicates the total articles by month that stated or implied that fear over BSE or CJD was unnecessary, neutral or valid. Figure 12.2 indicates these results graphically.

E. Assignment of blame

Results of analysis of the implication of British Government incompetence are shown in Tables 12.7 and 12.8. Table 12.7 indicates the number of articles by month that mention the competence of the Government. Table 12.8 indicates the per cent of total articles for that month. Many articles did not mention government competence and are not incorporated in this analysis.

Table 12.6 Average augmentation of fear, 1996

Month	Jan	Feb	Mar	April	May	June	July	Aug	Sept	Total
Unnecessary	1	0	6	26	10	4	25	8	2	82
Neutral	0	0	1	14	45	1	1	1	11	74
Augmented fear	6	9	94	55	15	32	4	17	37	269
Total	7	9	101	95	70	37	30	26	50	425

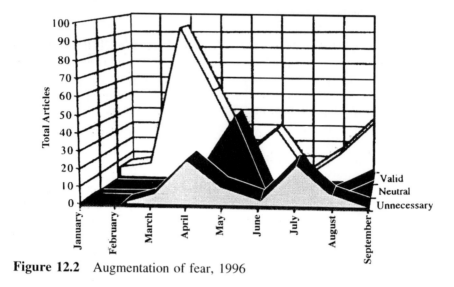

Figure 12.2 Augmentation of fear, 1996

Table 12.7 Implication of Government incompetence by month, 1996: raw number

Month	Jan	Feb	Mar	April	May	June	July	Aug	Sept	Total
Yes–explicit	0	0	14	6	9	3	4	2	6	44
Yes–implicit	0	0	15	26	12	2	5	3	8	71
No	0	0	4	2	0	1	1	0	1	9
No mention	7	9	68	61	49	31	20	21	35	301
Total	7	9	101	95	70	37	30	26	50	425

Table 12.8 Implication of Government incompetence: percentage of monthly total in 1996 (percentage of total articles, 425)

Month	Jan	Feb	Mar	April	May	June	July	Aug	Sept	% of Total
Yes–explicit	0.0	0.0	13.9	6.3	12.9	8.1	13.3	7.7	12.0	10.4
Yes–implicit	0.0	0.0	14.9	27.4	17.1	5.4	16.7	11.5	16.0	16.7
No	0.0	0.0	4.0	2.1	0	2.7	3.3	0.0	2.0	2.1
No mention	100.0	100.0	67.2	64.2	70.0	83.8	66.7	80.8	70.0	70.8

Discussion

Media analysis of BSE in the *Financial Times* indicates that: (1) the media filled a void and became the primary health disseminator, drawing conclusions regarding health risks; (2) the media engendered fear over BSE; (3) the media misinterpreted scientific data about BSE; and (4) the Government was portrayed as unreliable and incompetent in dealing with the BSE crisis.

A. Inaccuracy of media reports

The March 1996 BSE crisis generated several scientifically inaccurate articles in the press. When reporting the BSE issue, the press may have felt pressure to sensationalize and exaggerate the risks. George Parker, a journalist for the *Financial Times* stated, "There is no doubt that the scare was hyped up [in other publications]. Certainly that would be the instinct of most journalists – to hype the story up – rather than play a socially responsible (role) in relating issues."[5] The root of this pressure is derived from the nature of the popular press – namely, to sell papers. Nils Bruzelhius, health and science editor for the *Boston Globe*, said that in considering whether to print an article, "Ultimately, [a news editor] thinks about if the reader will be interested in an article" (8 January 1997). In an effort to attract readers, a dominant question for editors is whether to report unattractive issues that may not be desired reading, or whether to report issues that attract consumers.

Most notably, British newspapers misrepresented the health risks. The London *Times* article entitled "Call for watchdog as CJD toll hits 15" (Michael Hornsby, 7 January 1997) states, "15 people were so far believed to have fallen victim to a strain of Creutzfeldt–Jakob disease linked to eating BSE-infected beef." But, there had been no scientific evidence linking BSE to CJD. At best, there was only a theory that BSE could have "jumped the species barrier" and infected a human. SEAC specified that there is "no direct evidence of a link", and the suspicion of BSE causing CJD is due to the "absence of any credible alternative."[6]

Articles in the *Financial Times* inaccurately reported scientific data on BSE, particularly portrayal of a link between BSE and CJD. It was found that the reporting of the scientific interpretation of BSE was sometimes inaccurate in the early days of reporting after the Government's announcement, but became more accurate in subsequent weeks. The accuracy of articles was particularly clear in the representation of a "definite" link between BSE and CJD. In fact, there were five times as many articles that discussed "definite links" in March than in any other month. All of those articles appeared in only one week during March. Therefore, March had a concentration of articles discussing a "definite" link that was twenty times higher than the month with the next highest concentration of such articles. Fifteen articles in March discussed the "definite" link, ranging from headlines stating, "Mad cow disease linked to humans" (*Financial Times*, 21 March 1996), to articles that referred to "the link between bovine spongiform encephalopathy and the fatal human brain ailment Creutzfeldt–Jakob disease" ("Angry farmers blame Britain for price collapse", 29 March 1996).

However, some of these articles claiming a "definite" link also explained the link accurately. Often, *Financial Times* journalists were correct in their articles, but the copy editors creating the headlines exaggerated the risks. Journalists used phrases in the article such as the following to describe risk: "Is not absolutely proved" (*Financial Times*, 21 March, "Resistant protein particle causes disease") and "there remains no scientific proof" (*Financial Times*, 21 March, "Mad cow disease linked to humans"). However, these statements were buried under the headlines of the articles on the front page: "Mad cow disease linked to humans", and "Resistant protein particle causes disease." The front page headlines almost certainly had more impact on influencing public opinion than details within an article. According to the *Financial Times*' staff writers, the headlines are written by the copy editors with little or no input from the journalists. The article cited above, "Mad cow disease linked to humans", indicates one area where the reliability of disseminated information broke down. While journalists for the most part were well-informed of the probabilities of risk, this may not have been true for copy editors. In the case of the BSE crisis, well composed and technically faultless articles were sometimes advertised with a headline that was scientifically false and promoted public fear.

It is possible that a headline that conveys false information could cause more damage than information in an article. Although this study did not examine headlines, it is likely that the public eye caught the front page headline, "Mad cow disease linked to humans" more often than it scrutinized the content of the article that followed it. It is also possible that a reader might remember information in the headline rather than in the article. In this way, the small amount of inaccurate information presented in headline form could have had a larger effect on public understanding than accurate information provided in the text.

The representation of the link between BSE and CJD in the first few weeks identifies how the media can misreport important scientific information integral to the public's comprehension of the issue. Press analysis in the early days of the BSE crisis may have been the most significant in shaping public opinion. With widespread public distrust of the British Government, due to suspicions that it was withholding dangerous information for political manipulation, attention on media information was at a peak. Hence, press reports in these early days were crucial in affecting public perception. Inaccurate health information, therefore, likely augmented national and international concern about the safety of British beef.

B. Portrayal of the Government as untrustworthy

The British Ministry's ability to communicate health information effectively was undermined by a public view that the Government was incompetent. That

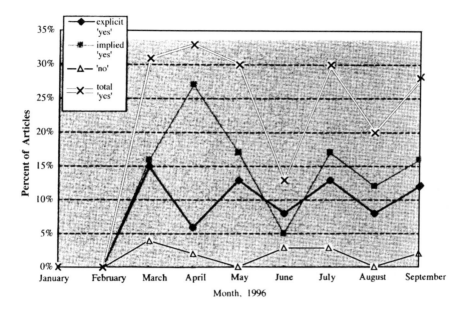

Figure 12.3   Expression of Government competence, 1996

does not implicate that the Government was not blameless. Disorganized and sometimes contradictory policies by the British Ministry, for example stances on cattle slaughter, EU conflict or co-operation, and international trade wars indicated that the Government was disorganized and in disagreement. Each political step was closely monitored and reported by the press. Indeed, a significant percentage of articles in the *Financial Times* stated or implied that the British Government was incompetent. However, in January and February, while governmental policy on BSE was secure and consistent, no article discussed the competence of the British Government. In fact, about one-third of *Financial Times'* articles between March and September commented on the government's incompetence in handling the BSE crisis. By contrast, only about three per cent of articles between March and September mentioned that the Government was not incompetent in its actions (see Figure 12.3).

C. The Press as the source of reliable information

During the BSE crisis, the media served as both information disseminator and risk assessor. In the early weeks of the crisis, there was a predominance of editorials on BSE in the *Financial Times*. While no editorials were published in January or February that mentioned BSE, even though there was speculated danger from BSE-infected beef, 17% and 15% of BSE articles were editorials in

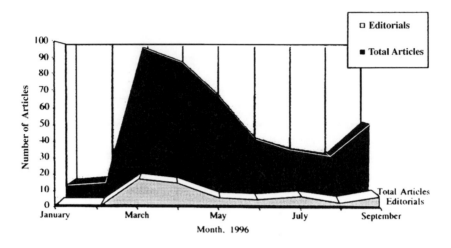

Figure 12.4 Total articles and editorials

March and April respectively. Subsequently, only 7% of the articles in May were editorials. Figure 12.4 shows the number of articles the *Financial Times* published by type.

The high percentage of BSE editorials in the initial weeks of the 1996 BSE crisis indicates that the press helped assess health information, (Mad cows and consumers, 27 March 1996), economic implications (The culling of Britain's cattle, 25 March 1996), and government mistakes (Livestock worries, 22 March 1996). The press therefore filled a void left by untrustworthy reports from the Government and unclear reports from the scientific community. However, there could not have been a concerted effort by all British journalists to convey risk accurately and uniformly. Hence, multiple versions of risk assessment predisposed the public to receiving multiple messages and potentially contradictory information. Contradictory information would confuse the readers further and probably lead to increased fear.

D. Contributing to the crisis

The analysis of whether articles promoted fear, had a neutral tone, or implied that fear was unwarranted, indicates that an overwhelming majority of articles contributed to the panic over BSE. Table 12.6 shows how each month except May had a predominance of articles that augmented fear. However, the articles are not slanted to inspire fear, in most cases the facts would tend to engender fear. Articles in January and February emphasize the tension over BSE when reporting on the British and German trade war (German States ban UK beef for BSE fear, 7 February 1996: 8) and economic hardship due to BSE effected sales

(Consumers still shunning beef, 31 January 1996: 10). March scandals that continued public hysteria included the Ministry's statement of BSE risks, the EU's response, individual country's positions, the worldwide ban on British beef products, and British citizen's fear of having eaten potentially contaminated beef. Most of the articles included dense facts and real news and lacked inflammatory wording which might have incited fear beyond what the facts themselves might have engendered. Some excerpts from articles are included below:

> McDonald's, the leading fast food chain, yesterday endured fierce questioning by MPs for leading the field in banning British beef from its restaurants because of the BSE crisis. (McDonald's accused of stoking public panic, 2 April 1996: 11)

> The government is likely to go along with farmers' refusal to accept the nationwide cull of cattle ordered by Brussels to stamp out BSE. (Hogg likely to seek selective beef herd slaughter, 6 April 1996: 4)

> Farmers are considering suing animal feed companies for negligence over the outbreak of the bovine spongiform encephalopathy epidemic. (Cattle farmers consider legal action over BSE, 11 April 1996: 8)

The announcement by Douglas Hogg on 20 March and the ensuing media frenzy begged closer examination of the true health risks of BSE. In the *Financial Times*, closer examinations appeared frequently two weeks after the announcement. Opinion pieces (including editorials and "op-eds" were categorized in this study as "editorials") printed from 21 March through 5 April augmented fear 94% of the time. However, editorials after 5 April augmented fear 24% of the time, were neutral 41% of the time, and stated or implied that fear was unwarranted 35% of the time. The raw numbers of editorials with different tones are shown in Table 12.9.

For example, the following article explained how fears over BSE were unwarranted.

> The interesting aspect of this [BSE] episode is the exaggerated reaction to very small risks – and indeed the inability or unwillingness of many so-called educated people to reason in terms of probabilities. Quick public judgments are often based not on any kind of risk assessment, but on what psychologists call the 'availability error' – that is, whatever first comes to mind. This in turn is determined by what has been recently publicized, sounds dramatic and can be expressed in images rather than abstractions. (Some ruminations on risk, Samuel Britain, 11 April 1996: 12)

Table 12.9 Tone of fear in editorials

Month	Augmented fear	Neutral	Fear unwarranted	Total
March	17	1	0	18
April	4	7	6	17

The famous video of cattle falling into walls and barking at people made the term "mad cow" an easily visualized image; but articles like Samuel Britain's began to publicly question the validity of BSE risks. The article headlined, "Government turns a drama into a crisis" (10 April 1996: 33), also addressed "the real, as distinct from the imagined, threat to health."

Note that these articles did not appear until three weeks after the beginning of the crisis. Why was there such a long lag time in publishing a more careful analysis of the health risks? The lag time could be due to the journalists not being specialists in scientific medicine or risk analysis. While this was Mr Hogg's duty, his influence was nullified by his political manipulation of the situation; but a journalist's responsibility is to report news without bias.

Assuming that there was unnecessary fear in the beginning of the BSE crisis, it appeared that responsible journalists stepped forward to curtail unnecessary fear. Unfortunately, lacking an organized body to assess health risk, journalists were without a reliable source to scientifically assess the issue and must rely solely on lay reasoning. A key question remains, however. Can a few well-reasoned articles published three weeks after the beginning of the crisis counter the fear generated by many more articles through the crisis peak?

Conclusion

The global fear of a relatively minor disease,[7] indicates that health risk information dissemination was at least partly to blame for the BSE crisis of 1996. It is evident that the British Ministry of Health as well as the scientific community made errors in communicating the risks. Both made public statements which misrepresented the risks or were unclear in their portrayal. The British media compounded the problem by making mistakes in health risk information dissemination. Analysis of the *Financial Times'* articles and editorials represented a consistent and conservative standard from which to judge the British media representation of BSE.

In the early days of the 1996 crisis, *Financial Times'* articles inaccurately described the scientific link between BSE and CJD, citing a definite link between the diseases at a relatively high frequency. Also during this period, opinionated editorials augmented fear at a high rate. The situation was exacerbated by the fact that *Financial Times'* articles portrayed the Government as incompetent in assessing the health risks and developing appropriate policy. The Ministry of Heath's ability to deal with the crisis was therefore undermined by a lack of trust.

Certainly the press' portrayal of the Government as incompetent was appropriate. First, it appeared that the British Ministry withheld reports discussing the dangers of BSE from the public. Because there was not immediate disclosure of the scientific reports by the Government, and the report was publicized first by the media, the Government appeared to be suppressing the information to avoid political embarrassment and economic crisis. Secondly, the Government's hasty reaction to the announcement, to which the EU was not given adequate warning, indicated that the British Government was unprepared and gave the appearance that the Ministry did not intend to publicize the information. Thirdly, the public statement issued by the Ministry did not explain the public health risks clearly. Fourthly, inconsistencies between Government statements eroded much of whatever credibility remained, and finally, contrasts between scientific and Government statements undercut the Ministry's reliability.

By withholding information, the British Government tried to protect the public from unnecessary fear. Instead, it created a crisis which fostered even greater fear.

The press eagerly filled the information void and fueled the crisis. Without a reliable central agency to disseminate trusted health information, the press presented inaccurate information and unsubstantiated conclusions. Fortunately, a few journalists gained perspective of the situation and published a fair portrayal of the risks, but not in time to alleviate the damage done in the previous weeks.

Notes

1 According to Alison Maitland of the *Financial Times* on 3 February 1997, the SEAC report was submitted to the Government days before any public announcement was made.

2 "Dorrell reassures over risks to children." *Financial Times*, 26 March 1996: 1.

3 "EU considers cash package to help all beef producers." *Financial Times*, 22 March 1996: 10. "4.5 million cows may face slaughter." *Financial Times*, 25 March 1996: 1.

4 Circulation information provided by the *Financial Times*. Daily circulation is based on September 1995 through February 1996 measurements.

5 28 January 1997. It is important to note that Mr Parker was not referring to the *Financial Times* and that the *Financial Times* firmly believes in reporting news without bias.

6 CJD Surveillance Unit. 3 February 1997.

7 It now appears that the new variants of CJD (v-CJD) may affect individuals. A

recent article in *Nature* states that, "It now appears that the case numbers (of CJD) really are going to get published from the Edinburgh group suggesting 'hundreds' rather than 'millions' of v-CJD cases. (vol **385**, 17.1.97, page 200) Furthermore, because the incubation period of CJD is so extensive, many people with these cases will die of other causes before v-CJD affects them."

Chapter 12, part iii

An Analysis of Media Coverage of the BSE Crisis in the United States

Veronica Demko

Introduction

The controversy surrounding BSE (bovine spongiform encephalopathy) holds many implications for the interface of politics, media, economics and health in the UK and the rest of the world. It is nearly impossible to discuss "mad cow disease" without taking into account not only scientific evidence, but also the political and economic agendas of the parties involved. Some of the stakeholders in this crisis include Government officials, who seek to protect the safety, prosperity, and support of their constituents; consumers, who want to protect their health and rights; scientists, who make projections and attempt to quantify risks; and media professionals, who attempt to inform the public while keeping interest levels high.

Usually the interests of these groups do not coincide, so it is difficult to create policies that satisfy everyone. In the case of mad cow disease, a public health issue became a political, industrial, and media issue. This phenomenon holds true for many other contemporary issues as well, including the silicone breast implant controversy currently underway in the United States, where FDA risk communication became interwoven with consumer fears and legal proceedings. Examining the ways in which BSE became a public issue can help us to understand how other health issues might find their way into the public.

The purpose of this study is to analyze the US coverage of the mad cow crisis and how political and media events in the United Kingdom and Europe were interpreted in the United States. In many cases, it becomes apparent that journalists suffer from opposing pressures: the complexity of the facts involved on one side, and readers' thirst for concise answers on the other. In addition, news accounts can only be as accurate as the news on which they report. The lack of effective communication and the simplification of facts which occurred on a political level, are reflected and propagated in the media coverage of this crisis. In order to present the situation to readers, reporters often choose to focus on a narrow aspect of the issue and use repeated narrative and metaphor to explain the situation to readers. This simplification may often be a reflection of journalists' own lack of understanding of the BSE issue, not necessarily an attempt to incite panic or distrust.

This analysis also studies the treatment that US newspapers give to any US threat of BSE or CJD (Creutzfeldt–Jakob disease). This can be assessed not only by looking at articles which focus on the US, but also on those that attempt to distance US readers from the crisis occurring in Great Britain by characterizing it as one that stems from British national identity.

Methodology

A content analysis was performed on articles from five major US newspapers: *New York Times, Chicago Tribune, Los Angeles Times, The Wall Street Journal* and *Washington Post.*[1] These newspapers were chosen because they are representative for circulation, population base, and ethos in the government and business sectors in the US. A search was conducted on Newspaper First Search, a complete database of over 25 daily newspapers, to identify all articles indexed by the terms bovine spongiform encephalopathy, mad cow disease, or Creutzfeldt–Jakob disease which appeared between 1 January and 1 November 1996.

The articles were coded according to the criteria in the Appendix. The coding system was tested by two evaluators on five randomly selected articles. An inter-rater reliability of 95% was established, and the system was used to analyze the remaining articles.

Results: Overview

Table 12.10 shows the types of articles that appeared in US newspapers. While the coverage of BSE in America included a wide variety of viewpoints and topics, some factors that emerged from the analysis were news articles, 105 (71 per cent); 90 articles (61 per cent) mentioned a possible link between BSE and CJD; most articles (70 per cent or 104 articles) did not refer to specific cases of CJD; 54 per cent of the articles examined focused on events in the UK; of 301 total quotes and references, 147 (49 per cent) were from government sources; and 84 per cent did not mention a potential threat to the US of BSE or CJD.

From these frequent factors, patterns begin to emerge among articles on the subject, which point to the power of the media in reflecting and shaping public perceptions of the mad cow crisis.

Table 12.10 Source of articles and type of coverage

	Number of articles	Per cent of total
Source of article		
New York Times	80	55
Chicago Tribune	22	15
Los Angeles Times	21	14
Washington Post	17	11
Wall Street Journal	8	5
Total	148	100
Type of coverage		
News	105	71
Analysis	20	14
Editorial	8	5
Letter	4	3
Humor	3	2
Other	8	5
Total	148	100

History of the BSE Crisis, as Reflected in US Newspapers

Many of the articles studied in this analysis focus on particular aspects of the crisis, such as the trade ban imposed on British beef products, or new scientific developments in BSE research. For the US readership, for whom BSE is not as widely understood as in Europe, many articles summarize the situation to form a context for the news story. An article in the 2 April 1996 *New York Times*, for example, entitled "Britain asks Europe to pay most of cost of killing cows", is concerned with the financing of Britain's culling plan, but it does give a brief history of the crisis:

> It was apparent that the [EU's] export ban would not be lifted any time soon. The ban was imposed after British ministers said that mad cow disease in cattle might be linked to cases of a fatal degenerative brain disease in humans.

Most articles that mention a "possible" link between BSE and CJD also focused on other aspects of the issue, but quote or refer to the 20 March 1996 announcement to give the context of the story. A 23 April 1996 piece in the *Washington Post* summarizes:

> The beef crisis here [in London] began March 20, when the government announced that a panel of scientists had concluded that

bovine spongiform encephalopathy, the cattle disease that has infected about 150,000 animals here over the past decade, was a 'likely' cause of a similar fatal brain disorder in humans, called Creutzfeldt–Jakob Disease.[2]

Discussions of Cases of CJD

In addition to frequent brief summaries of the 20 March 1996 announcement, 38 articles (26 per cent) mention the connection between BSE and particular cases of CJD. This number includes a wide range of articles among the papers: none of the articles in the *Wall Street Journal* mention the link between BSE and particular cases, while 30 of the articles in the *New York Times* do refer to this link. Thus, for most of the 72 per cent of articles which mention a link in general terms, no specific information is given as to the small number of people who have been diagnosed with the new strain of CJD.

Mad Cows and Englishmen

The *New York Times* reported on 7 April, in an article entitled "March 31–April 6; herd journalism" some of the "amazing coincidences" among headlines across America: Mad cows and Englishmen, *The New Yorker*, 8 April; Mad cows and Englishmen, *The Detroit News*, 2 April; Mad cows and Englishmen prevail, *The Washington Times*, 2 April; Mad cows and Englishmen: Europe panics over possibly deadly British beef, *The Washington Times*, 2 April; Mad cows and Englishmen, *The Economist*, 30 March; A scare story of mad cows and Englishmen: politics, press, profit motive combine to frighten the wits out of beefeaters, *Washington Post*, 28 March; Mad cows and Englishmen; disease panic: beef scare takes toll immediately, while knowledge takes years, *The Baltimore Sun*, 28 March; Mad cows and Englishmen, *San Francisco Examiner*, 27 March.[3]

More than a simple coincidence, these headlines reflect a trend in US newspaper coverage linking beef consumption, mad cow disease and England. Many of the articles analyzed in this survey (including many in the *New York Times*) focused on the history of beef in England, and pointed out the connection between British identity and beef consumption.

For example, "A steak in the heart of Britain", appearing in the *Washington Post* on 2 April, said that "apple pie is less American than blood-red meat is British." A *Los Angeles Times* (4 May 1996) article entitled "Mad cow ban strikes at heart of British identity" calls beef "a dish that is a cornerstone here [in London] of the national psyche." In a *New York Times* article on 30 March 1996, Colin Spencer refers to the "beef-eating chauvinism" which peaked in the eighteenth century, when "England became the most carnivorous country in Europe, with each person consuming 147 pounds of red meat each year."[4]

Table 12.11   Blame assigned to spread of BSE and spread of BSE-related panic

Type of blame	No. of articles	Per cent of total articles which assign blame (*n*=72)	Per cent of total articles (*n*=148)
Government cover-up	4	6	3
Incompetence	16	22	11
Lack of communication	10	14	7
Spread of BSE-contaminated feed	28	39	19
Multiple causes of blame	14	19	9
Total	72	100	49

BSE: Who Is at Fault?

Many analyses of the mad cow scare provide reasons for the spread of BSE or the spread of the public panic that characterizes the BSE crisis. By looking at these explanations, we are able to gain insight into another way journalists relay aspects of this complex political and public health issue for readers. Table 12.11 summarizes the reasons offered in US coverage for the BSE crisis.

One or more explanations for the BSE crisis were provided by 72 articles (49 per cent of all articles examined). Many of these explanations refer to the UK Government in some way: a cover-up, lack of communication between parties involved, or Government incompetence. Also, blaming the spread of BSE on the use of contaminated feed also indirectly blames the Government, since it reflects a lack of enforcement of feeding bans.

Sheep to Cows to Man: The Metaphor of a Food Chain Gone Mad

Of all the articles that assigned blame for BSE, 28 (39 per cent) state that the problem of BSE began when farmers began to feed rendered sheep to cows. In "A steak in the heart of Britain" (*Washington Post*, 2 April 1996), the author quotes an eighteenth century observer:

> It is that dreadful mixture of the souls ... of so many thousand animals, destroyed to pamper one, that raises that terrible war in the blood which as make it a prey to such distempers as have baffled the skill of the most learned physicians.

One prominent example of this concept is the diagram which appeared in the 1 April edition of *Health Journal* in *The Wall Street Journal*.[5] The diagram depicts a circle connecting a sheep, a cow and a man eating a hamburger.

The Harms of all Meat

In addition to many articles which address the problems of including meat in animal feed, there are some, like "Eating cows is the real madness" in the 9 April *Washington Post*, and "Vegeteens" in the 19 June *Chicago Tribune* which mention vegetarianism as a way to avoid contracting "mad cow disease" and other problems associated with meat eating. "Vegeteens" states that "while adults may fret about mad cow disease, saturated fatty acids ... and the effects of growth hormones, many American young people are swearing off meat altogether." "Eating cows is the real madness" states that the scare over BSE is an overreaction, but that eating a low-fat vegetarian diet is the way to avoid "heart disease, cancer, hypertension, diabetes, obesity and food-borne illnesses" which are some of the "medical blights directly associated with flesh-eating." In different ways, these journalists use BSE as a vehicle for discussing vegetarianism.

The Language of Mad Cow

Perhaps the most effective indication of what Americans have learned about the mad cow crisis is the description of the situation given in articles which are mainly unrelated to the topic, written by journalists other than those who normally cover the BSE situation. This can help to show how journalists themselves have learned from other media sources. Through these articles, we can begin to gauge the extent to which "mad cow" has entered the American vernacular, and see the values and assumptions which go along with this language.

In a 10 June 1996 *New York Times* feature entitled "In Japan, deflating a poisonous pufferfish legend", there is a small mention of BSE:

> Kiyoharu Hayashi, the head chef at Zuboraya, whose three outlets go through 4,400 pounds of pufferfish on a busy day, insisted that restaurant patrons face no danger. With a dig at Britain's problems with mad cow disease, he mused, "Maybe now fugu [pufferfish] is safer than hamburger."

Also in the *New York Times*, "Newt Gingrich, a vegetarian? Only in a prankster's dream", appearing in the 2 April 1996 issue, describes Gingrich's fake announcement of his switch to vegetarianism:

An official-looking statement purporting to be from Speaker Gingrich's office quoted the Georgia Republican as saying, "Don't have a cow; it's just a life style change." By way of further explanation, Mr. Gingrich admitted he was afraid of mad cow disease, which is making hash of Britain's beef industry but has not yet invaded North America.

The journalist once again breaks the mad cow issue down into more understandable parts, one of which is the assurance that Americans are safe from the disease.

Discussion

The articles appearing in major US newspapers usually include accounts of the UK Government's 20 March 1996 announcement of a possible link between BSE and CJD as a synopsis of the history of the mad cow crisis. This may reflect the fact that the announcement originally sparked the public controversy surrounding British beef. This announcement turned what had been viewed as a veterinary problem into a potentially human one. Most US coverage of BSE in 1996 (99 per cent, or 146 articles) takes place after the 20 March announcement, suggesting that the topic of BSE became newsworthy because of it.

Another factor that may have contributed to repeated synopses of the 20 March announcement is that journalists have a limited amount of space in which to fit news. A long history of the crisis would not be feasible in every news story. Also, for many readers who are familiar with the issues already, an extensive account of the complexities of the situation would be repetitive.

In spite of these journalistic reasons, however, the effect of "boiling down" the history of the crisis into a single sentence clearly omits important factors in the case, such as the degree of uncertainty involved in the announcement, the lack of conclusive data leading to it, and the controversy surrounding the decision to make the announcement. By choosing only to repeat the announcement itself, each article which describes another aspect of the crisis (i.e. the trade war, culling plans) serves to contribute to a sense of certainty surrounding the link to CJD by taking the "link" for granted.

Another significant trend in US coverage of BSE is the lack of specificity that accompanies each mention of a general "link" between BSE and CJD. While 72 per cent of all the articles examined mention a link, only 26 per cent give information as to the rarity of CJD. While a "link" is often assumed in many articles, the reader is left to guess at the extremely low incidence rate of CJD and the small potential risk for contracting the new variant.

This analysis of US coverage of BSE uncovered another journalistic trend, which is the connection often formed between "mad cows and Englishmen".

159

The authors of these articles, many of them British themselves, recognize the BSE crisis as one that threatens the foundations of England's identity, not simply due to the politics of the beef market, but because of the cultural and historical importance of beef in England. What becomes apparent in US newspaper coverage is that the effects of these articles combine to create the social construction of a link in American media between "mad cows and Englishmen". This image serves a useful purpose in American consciousness, which is to distance the American reader from the BSE crisis which occurs "over there". The more the diseased beef can be attributed to the UK, the lower the fears that it could become an American problem. Mad cow disease is depicted to derive from a national overindulgence in beef. The metaphor allows American readers to feel safe while blaming the seemingly stuffy, unnatural British traditions which have caused such problems. Many of these articles separate British beef problems from our own supposedly "healthy" consumption of beef.

In addition to discussions of national identity, reports of blame for the BSE crisis can also lend an insight into the workings of the press as mediator between government agencies, scientific sources, and the public. As mentioned earlier, over half of the total quotes originated from government sources. Since 21 per cent of all articles assign blame directly to the Government, and an additional 19 per cent blame the use of contaminated feed, the results suggest that many journalists, while reporting on government actions, are skeptical of the information they receive from government sources. This may reflect the public's distrust, and may also help to propagate it. Unfortunately, journalists had few other sources of information regarding mad cow disease. As examined earlier in this book by Catherine Goethals and colleagues (Ch. 9) there was no unbiased investigation of the situation: all sources had economic and political reasons to release the information they did. The US press reflects the confusion and distrust that characterized this issue from the beginning.

One source of blame attributed to the spread of BSE, including sheep parts in cattle feed, which is still a theory, makes for "excellent copy" in American newspapers. In Old Testament style, the unnatural practice of feeding meat to herbivores is seen to be delivered upon humankind in the form of CJD. While it may be beneficial for consumers to question the ingredients in cattle feed, it can be simplistic and even harmful to perpetuate the idea that such an easy and complete connection exists, through feed practices or any other link, without the evidence to support it.

This analysis also examines articles which do not focus on the BSE crisis, but which do make mention of mad cow disease, BSE, or CJD. Like articles about British identity, many of these unrelated articles also serve to distance the reader from BSE and CJD by assuring that Americans are not in danger of contracting mad cow disease, which often refers in these articles to both the bovine and human encephalopathies.

These articles reflect a fear of contracting mad cow disease by eating beef. Most journalists who report on the BSE issue itself are careful to separate BSE, or mad cow disease, and CJD, the disease in humans which is similar on a molecular level. In other sectors of reporting, however, the two diseases merge together into a menacing brain disease which is seen to be rampant in both cows and humans. On 28 March, the *Los Angeles Times* published a column entitled "A terminal case of mad GOP disease", which uses a metaphor of mad cows to describe the actions of California Republicans:

> there has been no recorded case of "mad cow disease" in the United States, but you wouldn't know it ... by watching ... GOP leaders stumble around in confusion.... They may not have been eating British beef, but for the last year they have been devouring their own.

In using the images of CJD (eating British beef) and BSE (stumbling in confusion) interchangeably, this column reflects an understanding of BSE as a disease that not only can be contracted by humans, but which manifests itself the same way in humans and cows. Once again, even though the topic is unrelated, the columnist reassures American readers that they are safe from this frightening, yet somehow humorous British disease.

Summary

The analysis of major US newspaper coverage of the mad cow crisis revealed several common frameworks for explaining the situation to American readers. While some journalists successfully conveyed the complexity of the issue and the conflicting interests of the stakeholders involved, almost all of the accounts of BSE and CJD in the study employed a strategy to "make sense" of the situation for readers, through a simplification of the facts of the crisis. This process of simplification is apparent in many newspapers' treatment of the history of the problem and the placement of blame for the situation. In addition, many articles served to assure the American public that BSE is a wholly British problem, either by linking beef to England's identity as a nation, or by reaffirming that there is no threat of BSE or CJD in the United States.

In the case of the mad cow issue, newspapers play a large role in helping the public form perceptions of the severity and likelihood of contracting CJD. In US newspapers, a wide variety of news events and opinions are represented about these issues. Thus the messages that reach a reader contribute either to that reader's sense of complacency regarding beef, to his or her fear of contracting CJD, or to the reader's level of understanding of the complex issues involved. These attitudes may shape consumer confidence in American beef, which in turn affects the market, politics, and the media.

It is also important to note the relationship between newspapers and the public. While the press does help to shape opinion, the media also receives its cues from the public. In the case of mad cow disease, the lack of trust in the Government, the lack of communication between the Government and scientists, and the lack of unbiased sources of information, all are passed on to the journalist and reflected in the stories written about the subject. It may be too easy to blame the media for the panic surrounding BSE. Rather, we should look deeper into the causes for the simplification apparent in press coverage, at the sources of information on which the media depended.

This content analysis helps to understand not only how a food scare is shaped by government, media and science, but also how mass media plays a large role in shaping public attitudes towards a very *public* health issue. In general, most major American newspaper coverage supposes a possible link between BSE and CJD, but separates American readers from the problem through reassurances or tying the problem to British identity. While it is true that American cattle may not be at risk of contracting BSE, there are other public health issues which are similarly shaped by the media. A look at the forces that shape media attention of the mad cow issue may help us to remain vigilant for future reports that attempt to "make sense" of complex aspects of our health, rather than giving us the tools to make sense for ourselves.

Notes

I am indebted to the editor, Dr Scott C. Ratzan, for suggesting this project to me and for offering his support and guidance throughout.

1 The data set used in this study also served as the basis for another manuscript, currently under review by an academic journal.
2 Britain threatens trade war. *Washington Post*. 23 April 1996: A12.
3 31 March–7 April 1996; herd journalism. *New York Times*. 7 April 1996: 4, 2.
4 The beef that built an empire. *New York Times*. 30 March 1996: 1, 23.
5 US groups move to make cattle feed safe for food chain. *Wall Street Journal*. 29 March 1996: A8.

Appendix: Criteria for Evaluating Articles

Type of article

News: A description of events.

Analysis: A description of a news situation, of other newspapers coverage, or a news piece which expresses an opinion without attributing it to a source (i.e. use of the word "should" or adjectives such as "incompetent", "biased", etc. without attribution).

Editorial: An opinion piece written by the editors of the newspaper.

Letter: A signed letter, or an op-ed piece. In the analysis of UK coverage, op-eds were classified as "editorials".

Humor: A piece which uses humor or "spoofs" the mad cow situation.

Non-BSE: An article that mentions BSE but is not based on the BSE issue.

Other: Any item not falling into one of the above categories. This could include cartoons, features, or corrections.

Primary setting of events

This refers to the principal setting of the article. The categories are:

UK

US

EU: The European Union as a whole.

Other: Includes countries outside of those mentioned above, as well as a particular country within the European Union.

Definition of link between BSE and CJD

No link: The article states that there is no link between the two diseases.

Possible link: A statement of a potential link. The language used in this statement could include: possible link, may be linked, believed to be linked, or suspected link.

Probably link: A statement that the link is probable, likely, or supported by evidence.

Definite link: A statement that there is no doubt that a link exists.

No mention: The article does not mention a link between the two diseases.

Cases: definition of link between the recent cases of CJD and BSE

The criteria and language are the same for the BSE-CJD link, but in reference to the link between BSE and specific cases of variant-CJD.

Quotes and references

The first three quotes or references in each article were coded according to the source.

Scientific community member: A medical doctor, researcher, or other scientist, or scientists in general.

Business community member: This category includes chairs or spokespersons of corporations, or those who analyze business data.

Government representative: This category includes elected officials as well as business people or others who are quoted as representing a Government agency.

General public: A consumer or other person whose occupation does not fall into one of the professional categories listed above.

Agricultural community member: This category includes farmers and ranchers, as well as representatives of farming or ranching associations.

Other: All other sources. These could include other newspapers, historians, poets and writers.

Assignment of blame

This refers to blame for the problem or problems which the article discusses. The categories are as follows:

No mention: The article does not assign blame.

Government cover-up: The article says that the UK Government did not share all the known facts with the public, and that this led to an escalation of the crisis.

Government incompetence: The article says that the UK Government made mistakes in handling the situation, or did not have the ability to handle the situation.

Lack of communication: The article states that risk was not communicated properly to the public by government or scientific sources.

Use of meat products in bovine feed: The article states that the reason for the BSE epidemic is the use of sheep and cow products in feed.

Multiple: The article says that more than one reason exists for the current situation.

Other: The article states a reason which does not fall into one of the above categories.

Subject

This category described the way in which the articles portrayed the BSE crisis. Five distinctions were made:

Scientific report: Article based on a scientific report on BSE or CJD.

Government wrangling: Articles directly attacking the UK Government's handling of the BSE issue.

Eurosceptic: Articles based on a Eurosceptic view of the European Union.

Plan of Government: Articles describing a plan of the Government in dealing with BSE as a disease, or the economic issues related to BSE.

Economic: Article which discusses the past or potential economic ramifications of BSE.

Part IV

Lessons and Possibilities

Chapter 13

Avoiding, Averting and Managing Crisis: A Checklist for the Future

Michael A. Chamberlain

In 1989, the Commons Agriculture Committee castigated the handling of the salmonella in eggs disaster as "a failure of government". The one certainty about the BSE catastrophe is that it merits that description, with a row of noughts on the end. (*The Daily Telegraph* 7 May 1996)

The mad cow disease issue was described by the Prime Minister of Britain (April 1996) as "the worst crisis a British Government has faced since the Falklands [War]". Even this rhetoric hardly did justice to the magnitude of the calamity.

It was not just a £550-million-a-year export industry which had been lost (perhaps never to be regained). It was not just the many thousands of jobs that had been lost, and the corresponding misery caused to farmers, slaughterhouse workers, butchers, and other work groups. It was the damage caused to European Union (EU) relations, which some commentators say will lead to the EC's (European Community's) eventual break-up, or at least Britain's withdrawal from its Continental trading partners.

Continued mishandling of the issue dogged the British Government's every move culminating in a parliamentary vote in September 1996 which the Government won by only one vote, thus preventing the inevitable vote of no-confidence which would have followed. It is this crisis in confidence in such an emotive area as public health issues, or rather the British Government's sorry handling of same, which may never be fully healed. As a lesson in inept communication the saga has few equals.

This book explores a plethora of ethical, political and health communication concerns on the mad cow issue and media coverage in detail. In particular, it looks for positive lessons to be learned for the future, and in this chapter I would like to stress that whether it be BSE, anti-smoking, screening for breast cancer, HIV or any preventative medicine campaign, a central policy which needs to be adopted is the dissemination of health messages *by all, relevant, available means.* Traditional mass communication vehicles, such as television and radio, although still powerful, need to be increasingly augmented by additional media which have become known collectively as "new media technologies". Health communication professionals need to learn that each medium has different properties and that some may be *controlled* more effectively than others with the result that the desired message can be retained intact.

The objective remains the use of effective communication to avoid or avert the crisis in the first place, but if, for whatever reason, crisis proportions have been reached, then that crisis must be handled – *managed* – until equilibrium can be restored.

Let us look at the range of media in more detail and, specifically, how emerging *new media* technologies may be harnessed more effectively in a crisis situation. Firstly, mass media: without government intervention on a massive scale, when draconian measures are deemed warranted, it is impossible to control the mass media. Blackouts do not work; ultimately, they are always broken. With mass media, the desired message is interpreted, diluted, commented upon, and distorted. The communicator can only hope that the message has been well prepared and placed in the right hands. Really? Even in the case of a nuclear catastrophe or warfare (the most readily proffered examples of situations requiring government intervention) no-one would claim that the Chernobyl Soviet nuclear reactor disaster was well handled from a communication point of view. And in warfare situations, the use of propaganda and disinformation techniques has so weakened the source to rule it virtually incredible.

The past few decades are littered with examples of the power of mass media overwhelming attempts at control: Vietnam, the Gulf War, Watergate, the list is substantial. In the political arena, attempts by "spin doctors" are undergoing increased scrutiny leading to ever less powerful results. The mass media remain in control; it is their massage if we can be forgiven for deliberately misappropriating the writings of Canadian communications guru Marshal McLuhan.

By contrast, let us examine new media technologies where the entry costs are much lower and where control – or at least elements of control – can be maintained. Electronic bulletin boards, closed user group messaging over intranets, hypertext-linked information available on internet world wide web sites, audiotext information lines, confidential electronic counselling by e-mail, and sound and video bytes stored digitally for replay and access are the platforms of tomorrow which allow the communicator better control on individual messages. What is even better these platforms are available today.

It may help us to understand these technologies if we look at the origins of so-called new media and the properties that make them different to traditional mass media.

The background lies in the convergence of computers, telecommunication, and multimedia content, delivered initially to the personal computer but, increasingly, heading for the television set, which itself is becoming a computer in its own right.

Although important, it is a side issue whether it is *two* technologies – Computer + Telecommunications – or *three* (to include the TV), which will shape these information super highways. In the foreseeable future at least, in *business* information will be sent/received on computers and at *home* they will be increasingly sent to the TV set mediated via cable, digital satellite, coaxial cable, fiber optics, cellular or other distributive means.

Along the way, the home market will go through a transitional period where information is ported to Personal Computers but the end game will be one black box (let's call it C-TV, the computer-television set), which will be the platform for all manner of multimedia and online applications, including the Internet.

In 1996, Philips, the Dutch electronics group, announced a set-top box to bring the "Net to the TV", priced at $289. Oracle, Mitsubishi, Olivetti, Acorn, Sony, and others, are launching Network Computers, priced at around $500 (or less) for the 1997 Christmas market, and, without dwelling on the debate between Larry Ellison, Oracle's CEO, and Microsoft's Bill Gates, who favors the "fat" software-loaded computer, let's just agree that the convergence of PCs and TV technology is already happening.

These changes in technology are having a profound effect *on the way in which people communicate* (at home and in the workplace) and we need to understand these changes, as communicators (health communication professionals or otherwise), if we are to manage information technologies effectively and optimize their use.

In essence, we are moving from the "age of mass communication" into a "new media era of interactive communication".

There are four features which characterize this new media age:

(a) *Demassification*; the increasing ability of consumers to go à la carte and choose from a whole smorgåsbord of media and information items, whether they are delivered by satellite, copper twisted wire, coaxial cable, fiber optics, or cellular. We could even include print here as a medium, but the issue still remains: will it be previewed or sampled electronically first?

(b) *Interactivity*; the ability of the receiver to "talk back" or interact with the information provider, at his or her own pace, and on areas that person wants to read/view/listen to, consume if you like. Technology is facilitating this process whether it be through hypertext links in the case of a computer (the ability to jump from one topic to another simply by clicking on an electronic button), or audiotex in the case of telephony, even confravision, which is a medium that will soon come very much into its own and will revolutionize the way in which we communicate.

(c) The third characteristic is *asynchronicity* (perhaps more easily understood as time change) which refers to the increasing ability of consumers to choose when to receive (or *not* to receive a particular message). Video cassette recording and e-mail are the best two examples of this phenomenon, and it is worth noting that, as a result, the sender (the information provider) no longer fully controls the message – the receiver, assuming he/she wants to download it in the first place can manipulate that message, listen/view part or all of it, change it, add/subtract to it, and send it to someone else with the initial information provider having virtually no "say" in the matter.

(d) The final characteristic is *mechanamorphism* (taken from the writings of Marshall McLuhan) which simply means that the medium changes the message. For example, e-mail is written in a different, much more intimate and casual way than a formal business letter.

A further point to remember is that the pace of these changes is accelerating. The telephone took 44 years to reach a 35 per cent penetration level among US homes, radio took seven years, television six years and the VCR, only four. But the age of computers – and the birth of the interactive communications era (the one we are in now) – is the area where change can truly be measured in nanoseconds. Look at the amazing growth of the Internet: in 1990 there were fewer than five million users worldwide; in 1996 most estimates put the figure in the US alone at 18 million with over 40 million users worldwide.

We've come along way from the first ENIAC megacomputer and the statement that all the world would ever need is six just like them!

The issue, therefore, for health professionals is how can you best harness these new technologies, which ones should you use, and when should you use them? Irrespective of selection, however, one must remember that the message remains paramount. Garbage In, Garbage Out is still an accurate reflection of digitized content. The cardinal rule must remain formulating the *right message*, to the *right people* by the *right means* (increasingly interactive media, which will be sought by individuals because of the powerful added value of being able to "talk back" to the source). This, coupled with the fact that you, the communicator, can manage your own messages, load them digitally for electronic transfer, and amend them as latest information dictates, makes the choice of new media particularly powerful.

Let's look at it from the perspective of the announcement of the feared spread of mad cow disease to humans.

In what can only be viewed as a misjudged strategy, the announcement was made by the Health Minister in the House of Commons under the guise that it *had* to be announced in the British parliament first (on constitutional grounds) before any communication to the EC or other interested parties. However, this entirely begs the question of how simultaneous messaging could be achieved or what additional channels of communication could be harnessed.

An ill-prepared and ill-equipped British parliamentary press corps were fed a story of impending doom with no thought of how the ensuing crisis could have been avoided, averted or, at the very least, managed. It should be remembered that British parliamentary proceedings are covered live by television.

A look at the headlines tells the whole sorry saga of allowing mass media alone to run with the story: Bad moos for Britain – Sales plunge as experts warn: That pub sandwich could be deadly, *Daily Star* 22 March 1996; Don't risk eating beef, *Daily Express* 23 March 1996; Chemical link to mad cow – Experts says BSE not caused by feed but pesticide, *Scottish Daily Express* 6 April 1996); No stopping beef panic, *Daily Express* 26 April 1996; Death sentence – Doctor says girl got human form of mad cow disease through eating burgers, *Scottish Daily Express* 27 April 1996; Slaughter of the mad cows, *Daily Express* 27 April 1996; Jobs slashed in beef crisis, *Daily Express* 2 May 1996; No method in this madness, *Daily Telegraph* 7 May 1996; Farmageddon – "Doomsday" warning on mad cow disease, *Daily Star* 22 May 1996; Bosses roast Tories over Euro-beef row, *Daily Express* 6 June 1996.

Imagine a more controlled set of announcements whereby mass media and new media were separately targeted.

(a) *Mass communication*: television, radio, press, posters, cinema, below-the-line (leaflets, "information" displays at health centers, schools, etc.). Managed communication messages could have included:
  (i) full fact briefings to specialist medical correspondents of the mass media (briefed in advance of the parliamentary announcement on an embargoed basis);
  (ii) pre-arranged television and radio interviews with informed experts (medical/scientific/agricultural);
  (iii) video and audio sound bytes recorded earlier and available for distribution to all mass media.
(b) *New media communication – information on demand*: electronic databases, bulletin boards, the Internet (and closed-user group intranets); e-mail, fax, fax-on-demand, audiotext, voicemail; interactive television, interactive kiosks, videotext (teletext), confravision (on demand); video and audio sound bytes; and, if appropriate, diskette, interactive video disc, CD-I, CD-ROM, CD-EROM, etc. Messages would include:
  (i) Information "hotlines" accessing databases by telephone (audiotext), fax (interactive fax services), e-mail (interactive or downloadable extracts, public statements, research findings, fact sheets, etc.), and, where appropriate, personal caller (health centers or specially organized personal response units where the response/degree of hysteria demanded it);
  (ii) electronic bulletin boards (with hypertext links to Internet sites);
  (iii) a National Health Service/Government Internet www site with hypertext links to other relevant sites and e-mail facilities for specific or "unanswered" questions;
  (iv) Briefing packs for journalists, farmers, medical staff, international access, etc. (available initially electronically for downloading or self-printing, but as time permitted, this would be augmented by print

press "advertisements", television/radio "infomercials", leaflet drops at medical centers, hospitals, etc.);

(v) separate closed user medical/agricultural briefings/seminars for relevant professionals encrypted for access pre-screened or via some type of available on-screening mechanism (for health communication issues, it is not unrealistic to amass regularly updated lists of personnel to be notified electronically or who have electronic access).

These communication channels could have been managed to address the fundamental issues: Can humans catch mad cow disease? Is there a link with CJD? What can be done to prevent it?

In the case of BSE, it is perhaps too late to put the clock back; but we can learn through our mistakes. We would all accept that the whole matter could have been handled better. A way forward would be to remember that when the next health crisis looms, reliance on mass media is an unacceptable risk. All technologies – including digital new media – can be harnessed to better effect, and digital dissemination of information is faster, more immediate, and more controllable than traditional mass media outlets.

Chapter 14

Farming with Nature: A Solutions-Oriented Strategy

Dawn Hopkins and Marcie Everett-Weber

The BSE Crisis and its Origins

The Common Agricultural Policy (CAP) was created in the 1950s as a post-war measure aimed at assuring a fair standard of living for the agricultural community. As a result, farming methods became too intensive, industrialized, and production-oriented, and carried significant risks for consumers and farmers.

In addition to this unhealthy premise of production-based farming, the British Government neglected early indications and warnings by independent scientists and took into account only the more reassuring opinions of scientists dependent on the beef industry. By championing deregulation, the British Government risked its citizens' health instead of adequately informing them and taking necessary preventative safety measures.

Originating from within a culture of outdated agriculture policies and spurred on by government inefficiencies, BSE became an issue of crisis proportions. As a result, consumer confidence eroded, the beef industry was decimated in the UK, beef sales plummeted throughout Europe, political and scientific sectors were rewarded with serious consumer distrust, and the economy received a significant set-back.

New CAP Objectives

The current direction of the CAP favors intensive, modern, mechanized systems and high production which result in crises such as the BSE scare. Today's European citizens, farmers, consumers, rural communities and environmental organizations have new needs and a modern vision of our rural environment. "Farming with Nature" is an agricultural movement spearheaded by the European Policy Office of the World Wide Fund (WWF EPO) for Nature in Brussels, Belgium. Farming with Nature seeks to promote and realize the main objectives for sustainable agriculture and rural development policies to result in healthy food in a healthy environment for all European citizens.

Farming with Nature and its supporters believe that a revised agricultural policy oriented towards new objectives would result in a more effective integration of agricultural, rural, and environmental concerns at all levels of policy implementation. It would thus provide new perspectives for sustainable agriculture and rural development in Europe for the twenty-first century.

A CAP based on more progressive objectives would offer the European agricultural sector a wider set of economic opportunities, recognition of their multiple functions, and thus a better chance of achieving equitable standards of living. Most importantly, new CAP policies could avert a crisis of the proportion of the BSE affair from occurring in the future.

Intensive Versus Extensive Farming

The critical consequences of intensive meat and milk production must be considered when questioning the devastation brought about by the mad cow crisis. Over the past 400 years intensive farming production has degraded or destroyed many of the world's ecosystems, impoverished the land and shortened the lives of humans. Today, across the globe, including Europe, pastures and landscapes have been destroyed by intensive meat producers and their crowded herds. The modern livestock economy has seriously altered the landscapes of our planet.

Intensive farming, with its emphasis on animal confinement and food supplements, has provided the model for conditions that generated mad cow disease in the UK. The overall industrial trends of these outdated farming practices include larger and larger corporate units, intensive methods of beef and milk production, protein supplements and growth hormones; a list of factors contributing to BSE.

Suggested Solutions and Recommendations for the BSE Crisis

The following recommendations are included to serve as a model of measures that should or already have been implemented to aid in the reduction and depletion of BSE contributing factors. This list is not necessarily endorsed by the WWF EPO, it merely serves as a paradigm for future crisis communications endeavors associated with BSE.

Steps to eradicate BSE

(a) A ban on the production and use of all meat meal in animal feedstuffs;
(b) a total ban on the use of diseased animal cadavers for animal feedstuffs, human nutrition and other forms of human consumption (i.e. cosmetics, medicines);

(c)　mandatory and precise labeling by the producers of industrial feedstuffs detailing complete information on the composition and origin of their products;

(d)　establishment of a publicly accountable scientific body, independent of the beef industry to monitor the situation, make recommendations and implement appropriate measures;

(e)　the development of effective and accurate tests for BSE detection;

(f)　culling of herds of diseased animals;

(g)　cull of all animals born before the ban on meat meal (1989);

(h)　ensuring safe standards of discharge for the effluent (blood and bodily fluids) remaining from the current culling process;

(i)　environmentally safe and effective removal and disposal of the remaining thousands of tonnes of contaminated animal feedstuffs;

(j)　new CAP policies encouraging a shift from intensive to extensive farming methods to halt further infection and spread of BSE.

Steps to rebuild consumer confidence

In the effort to restore consumer confidence, the previous recommendations should be reviewed in addition to the following actions to aid in rebuilding consumer confidence:

(a)　the identification of origin of all meat sold to consumers;

(b)　responsible communications to the public;

(c)　proof of action steps by the Government to ensure future public health safety;

(d)　all related information should be readily accessible to the public;

(e)　vendors must certify beef and beef products to meet the criteria of quality, value, safety, welfare and taste;

(f)　a shift away from intensive agricultural practice and towards sustainable agricultural and agricultural reforms.

Steps to reform the sector toward extensive farming

A large part of the western European agricultural surface encompasses favorable natural conditions for grasslands ideal for beef production. The diversity of soils, climate, bovine races, expertise, and local traditional beef products are a European wealth to be preserved, utilized, and promoted. However, Britain's Government and the agricultural industry have resisted calls from environmentalists and others to implement sustainable agricultural and other progressive reforms. The following proposals are suggested:

(a)　establishment of subsidies, tax breaks and incentive programs to encourage farms to shift toward more extensive farming methods;

(b) implementation of a supply management policy to maintain market price and to avoid dumping of surpluses;

(c) encouragement of beef production based on grazing to produce quality meat (grazing is obligatory for suckler cows and cattle older than 14 months during the period of grass growth. Grazing is not obligatory for cattle younger than 14 months in regions where grasslands are too scattered to allow for grazing).

(d) feedstuff must be appropriate for ruminants; at least 70 per cent of the feed must come from the farm, 30 per cent maximum can be purchased from outside sources in which preference should be given to the surrounding region. Concentrated feed must be European;

(e) rule of maximum stocking rate per hectare which will vary from region to region to protect underground water and soil.

Proposals to current CAP framework for beef reforms

In order to encourage extensive, sustainable agriculture and ensure sustainable living practices, CAP reform must be a priority. The following list of reforms are to be considered:

(a) a ceiling on farm supports (European and national);

(b) implementation of import tariffs and supply management policies to preclude the import of beef under the price of 4.1 green Ecu per kilo carcass;

(c) a ban on the use of meat meal in feedstuffs for animal production;

(d) a total ban on any growth promoters;

(e) a ban on all antibiotics mixed into feedstuffs;

(f) precise labeling on feedstuffs;

(g) replacing headage payment by hectare payment with appropriate environmental conditions attached;

(h) reducing the rigidity of livestock quotas on environmental grounds;

(i) assisting grazing of seasonal high mountain pastures through a shepherding allowances;

(j) CAP instruments which encourage farmers to introduce livestock into low intensity dryland systems, to improve soil structure, and create permanent pasture, thus reinstating mixed farming.

Proposals for farmer compensation

Farmers must be compensated for income losses this year and for the years to come as they shift to and integrate safer and environmentally sound farming standards. Compensation must be implemented during an adaption period to ensure the livelihood of farmers. One detrimental aspect of the current subsidy system is that intensive farming, which uses the most fertilizer and artificial aids for production, is the highest rewarded. Subsidies for intensive farming encourage the use of unnatural methods to boost production resulting in problems such as the BSE crisis. WWF's Farming With Nature, along with other organizations, recommend switching subsidies from production-based farming to environmentally safe and healthy farming. Subsequently, reverting to natural methods will help to ensure the goal of safer foodstuffs.

Costs for compensation should be shared by the UK (for not reacting more quickly and more prudently to the early signs of the crisis), by the European Union (for its outdated and unsound CAP), and by the agribusiness industry, specifically feedstuff manufacturers (for reaping billions in profits by recycling cadavers to produce meat meal which lead to the BSE crisis). Compensation includes and is not limited to:

(a) subsidies for extensive farming (not to exclude: switching subsidies from intensive based farming to extensive farming);
(b) tax breaks for extensive farming;
(c) reward programs for extensive farming.

Conclusion: Solutions for a Safer Future

Farming with Nature provides the guidelines for an environmentally and socially responsible agricultural policy to prevent future public health crises and to ensure sustainable living. Yet, the current direction of the CAP favors intensive, modern, mechanized systems and high production. At the same time, the European Union has an excess of agricultural products, which can result in crises such as that associated with BSE.

There are some voluntary schemes to encourage environmentally sensitive farming, but these are generally small and localized, and not always aimed at key areas. They support specific management practices but do not address the fundamental problem – the economic framework provided by the CAP.

British agriculture lags behind much of the European Union with one of the smallest percentages of land under organic production: only 0.3 per cent of British holdings are farmed organically. Reports of an increased interest in healthy farming practices underscores the British public's loss of confidence in British beef farming and industrial agricultural practices. Vegetarianism is gaining popularity and more people are turning to organic farming for solutions. According to John Vidal, environmental expert, "If the British Government wanted to restore the confidence in British agriculture, it would drop its hostility to sustainable, low intensity farming and subsidy procedures to turn organic. BSE makes us consider whether we can continue abusing nature and treating it as an infinite resource to tinker with" (Leech 1996).

Examples of Successful Extensive Practices

Britain appears somewhat interested in "green" farming methods following the BSE crisis while other member states have seen almost explosive growth in this sector. Generous taxpayer subsidies, concerned consumers and the Alps have made Austria the developed world's leading organic farming nation. Sweden follows in second place with 3.3 per cent of its farmland given over to organic production. Germany is third with just under 2 per cent.

Sweden's farmers are also proud of their attitude to the environment and animal welfare. The change in direction away from the most intensive methods, fostered by a mix of voluntary agreements and governments policies, began in 1953 when a salmonella epidemic killed 100 people.

In 1990, the Austrian government offered farmers new subsidies – for each hectare farmed according to strict organic and animal welfare principles, they would receive a fixed payment. The subsidies range from 3,000 schillings per hectare for organic grassland to 10,000 schillings for vines.

Another strand in Austria's environmental success story is the co-operation between organic farmers' associations and retailers which led to several main supermarket chains heavily backing organic produce. The subsidies started before Austria joined the European Union and have continued since CAP regulations allow them, but only as part of a "agri-environment" package subject to financial limits.

Britain only offers subsidies for the process of converting from intensive to organic production, but the uptake has been disappointing with only 0.3 per cent of agricultural land organically farmed. On a positive note, the 1000 select farms of Marks and Spencer (M&S) in Britain are following the principles of extensive farming. M&S cows feed on grass in the spring and summer and on silage (dried fermented grass) in the winter. This traditional feed is no more expensive than buying feed concentrates. Mr Gilbert Wood, technical manager for M&S points out, "It doesn't cost more to be a good farmer than a bad farmer" (Bateman 1996). Studies of Western European consumers indicate a growing demand toward organic food for safe consumption.

"Greens", better known as environmental supporters in the European Parliament, have argued that the mad cow problem is a product of "expert driven industrial farming methods that entail cheap production-boosting devices with unforeseeable consequences." Green representative Friedrich Wilhelm Graefe zu Baringdorf comments: "Consumer confidence can best be restored by regional markets in high quality meat raised in ways that are good for farmers, for the environment and for the animals themselves" (Leech 1996).

Gail Murray, campaigner for extensive farming with WWF International brings the issue into sharp focus: "British farmers are quite capable of producing wholesome and environmentally sustainable products. Agricultural policies must be changed to reflect this. Livestock policies must be reformed to promote quality not quantity" (WWF 1996).

Extensive or organic farming will not only meet these growing consumer desires, but also help to eradicate BSE, restore consumer confidence, and prevent similar public health and economic disasters in the future.

References

Bateman, M. 1996. "Keeping the carnivore satisfied". *Independent On Sunday*, 2 June: 56-60.

Leech, C. 1996. "Mad cows shake up British agriculture". *Alternatives Journal*, October–November **22**: 4.

WWF 1996. "Farming with nature objectives". *Farming With Nature Programme Strategic Planning Workshop Report*. 24 April. La Ferme de Froidmont: Belgium.

Chapter 15

Strategies for Attaining Public Health

Scott C. Ratzan

"They say" is the monarch of this country, in a social sense. No one asks *"who* says it," so long as it is believed that *"they* say it." Designing men endeavor to persuade the public, that already "they say" what these designing men wish to be said, and the public is only too much disposed blindly to join in the cry of "they say ..."

Every well meaning man, before he yields his faculties and intelligence to this sort of dictation, should first ask himself "who" is "they," and on what authority "they say" utters its mandates. (James Fenimore Cooper 1831)

While the educated "public" receive medical and health information that is disseminated through 25,000 scientific/medical journals throughout the world, most of us get the vast majority of our health information from popular media sources. Everyday, as we flip through the pages of newspapers, listen to the radio on the way to work, read billboards on the highway, thumb through magazines, or "surf" the hundreds of available channels on television or pages on the world wide web, we are bombarded by a subtle and not so subtle montage of health messages.

Simultaneously we encounter newscasts each day on radio and television informing us about the latest "discoveries" by scientists from throughout the world. Some of this information is pre-determined in the form of paid advertising. Some is quasi-planned – late breaking news. Yet, the product of this message mosaic is our mediated reality. Such data – scientific as well as "scientistic" – floods the secondary and tertiary wave of discussion within the public. Information evolves into accepted truth without real verification. Information becomes fact – the "stuff" of public discourse without real verification. In remembering Cooper's warning, "they say" takes on its own significance becoming the ethos, the common terminology and foundation from which our reality flows.

Today, over 25,000 scientific/medical journals publish studies annually, yet the public continues to receive as much as 85 per cent of health information from non-medical sources (Wilkes, 1997). Hence, the public knowledge of science is based primarily on how non-experts present it. The product of this process is that spurious speculation is confused with scientific fact. The conduits to the public's understanding of scientific issues are not the scientists, but politicians and self-anointed "experts" in the media.

The channels of traditional and new media present an opportunity to utilize an omnipotent venue through which millions of people at any given moment can gather and send information. Suffice it to say, these channels of communication provide unmatched opportunities to advance knowledge and our public health goals.

While the media is the primary disseminator of information used to improve public health, its ethical and efficacious operation is dependent, as is always the case, on its source and its credibility. To follow the media blindly is similar to naïvely depending on the public works system to provide a specific, exact road for you from your door to desired destination. Such expectations are simplistic, lacking the specifics of *where* you want to go, *how* you and your guests might travel (a bicycle, motor bike, van or car) and *why* you want to get there, invites one to be a victim of chance. Although it is easy to find a road, the simplest path does not always get you to your destination or produce the best intended result; you need to take charge of your journey.

The purpose of this chapter is to discuss effective strategies on effective communication of health – using our road analogy, our ability to accomplish the goal of getting from point a to point b – from sender to the specific and desired receiver. The exigence of the beef crisis in Europe provides a case for analysis. This chapter presents four perspectives commonly employed by the health communication strategist. Application of these approaches to the mad cow incident offers practical and heuristic understanding of not only the successes and failures plaguing this issue, but also a better appreciation of such orientations. Following a discussion of the theoretical precepts of such theories and a review of certain areas within health communication, an application of the BSE/mad cow crisis will be presented. Afterwards, questions in preparation of the best strategy to avert such a crisis in the future will be presented along with potential approaches.

The Case

The mad cow crisis of 1996 presents a provocative case for such a comprehensive analysis. For the purposes of this analysis, a brief descriptive background is provided.

Mad cows were first identified and named as such in 1986 following the pathological diagnosis of bovine spongiform encephalopathy (BSE) with the presumed infectious agent of a prion. The source of the emerging epidemic was presumably traced to a food supplement that included meat and bonemeal from dead sheep. The British Government banned the use of animal-derived feed supplements in 1988, a time identified as the epidemic's peak.

A similar brain disease on a molecular level, Creutzfeldt–Jakob disease (CJD) in contrast, occurs worldwide in humans and usually presents as dementia. Most of the time it appears sporadically, striking one person in a million annually, typically around age 60. Ten to 15 per cent of cases are inherited, and a few are iatrogenic – inadvertently spread through surgical or medical intervention by the attempt to treat some other problem.

A decade since the discovery of mad cow disease, a British Government report in March 1996 suggested mad cow disease could be transmissible to humans. The ensuing media frenzy crippled the British beef industry and further questioned the safety of the food supply throughout the world. It escalated to "the biggest crisis the European Union had ever had", according to European Commissioner for Agriculture, Franz Fischler. Later, a ban on British beef products was proclaimed by the European Union. In response, the British blockaded all European Union legislation and threatened to leave the European Union, effectively shutting it down for nearly two weeks. While the politicians argued long-term policy, UK and Swiss ranchers felt the impact of the initial response of the Government as their beef herds were untimely culled through Government directives, while the demand for the remaining beef diminished throughout Europe.

The mad cow issue is rooted both in the credibility of the Government releasing a questionable report, and the media creating and proclaiming the report as if it were factual in every way. In the mad cow case, the global interest and high drama simplified the press's job to report rather than to question adequately the veracity of the claims. Acting simply as disseminator, few challenged the questionable claim in a serious manner.

In the absence of an adequate campaign or co-ordinated, persuasive strategy to combat such a public frenzy, there was an absence of cogent decision making and public understanding based on verifiable fact. Nobody would accept responsibility to explain the crisis.

Context and Communication Strategies

As a conscientious health communicator, it is imperative to examine, understand and finally to act within the context of the entire situation – the large, macro-level as well as within the multiple, micro-levels of activity. In surveying the rhetorical landscape one must know: What strategies and mechanisms exist that can deliver appropriate information from sender to receiver?

In our road analogy it is important to know the map – the terrain, the quality and destination of the roads and highways. The challenge is to choose the best vehicle to negotiate within the crowded environment in the quest to reach the final destination. In health communication, the *map* can help us advance the public's knowledge about potential health hazards in the most efficient/efficacious way.

The different approaches outlined in this chapter have great potential, as they can each individually be more effective than the simple reliance on gut feelings, or the *laissez-faire* attitude frequently evident among the public-at-large. Each requires strong ethical responsibilities, by both the sender and the receiver of information.

Theoretical Overview of the Role of Communication

Any cogent communication strategy requires the identification of the essentials of communication: source, credibility, accessible and effective communication channels, message design, and audience characteristics. To be of heuristic and practical value, communication, persuasion, and behavioral theories should be employed with the knowledge of the social, political, economic and cultural constraints, and sustained for a sufficient period so as to promote understanding and long-term behavior change effectively among the targeted public.

Traditional linear communication models such as Shannon & Weaver (1949), and Lasswell's 1972 paradigm (Who/Says What/To Whom/In What Channel/With What Effect), established an important academic base for communication's development as a discipline. However, application of complex and dynamic communication models can further advance knowledge, understanding, interpretation and the pattern of the communication process. Linear models are: "... defined as the process by which messages are transferred from a source to a receiver. Such a one-way view of human communication describes certain types of communication; many kinds of diffusion do indeed consist of one individual informing another" (Rogers & Kincaid 1981: 63).

Yet, the process of diffusion of information throughout society is arguably more vividly explained through convergence models. Such models define communication as "a process in which the participants create and share information with one another to reach a mutual understanding" (Rogers & Kincaid 1981: 63).

As most health communication messages can be developed amongst the general umbrella terms of theories of rhetoric and communication – e.g. persuasion theory, exchange theory, and behavioral theory – an understanding of these areas is of paramount importance for the health communicator in any strategic orientation.

Theories of human behavior (e.g., social cognitive theory; Bandura 1986) and the processes of communication (e.g., network-based diffusion of innovations; Rogers 1983) enable health communicators to predict, explain, and prescribe strategies for influencing health behaviors at individual, dyadic, social network, organizational, and societal levels of analyses. Accordingly, different health communication messages targeted at each of these levels provide an interesting context of behavioral theories in the effort to interpret and predict behavior.

Exchange theory posits that health communication involves a voluntary exchange of resources (Lefebvre & Flora 1988). An effective health communication message viewed as a product or service that can bartered by both the buyer and the seller would exemplify an exchange application. To induce a response among audience members, such messages must provide important benefits of adopting health promotion or disease preventive behaviors that clearly outweigh the costs of "purchase" (adoption).

Individual level theories, such as social learning (Bandura 1986), expectancy (Ajzen & Fishbein 1980), information processing (McGuire 1989), risk behavior (Witte et al. 1996), fear appeals (Janis & Feshbach 1953), decision making (Kahneman & Tversky 1972), and negotiation (Fisher & Ury 1981), also can be useful in informing specific publics about health issues. Organizational level theories focus on the diffusion of innovations through networks of organizations (Zaltman & Duncan 1977). Societal level theories, such as agenda setting (McCombs & Shaw 1972), study the influence of mass media on what people ultimately determine as important, applications of agenda setting in health communication (Dearing & Rogers 1996) ultimately focus on how media coverage of the health (both risks and policy) has helped to direct public attention and heightened an issue for the public policy agenda consideration (Payne et al. 1989). Given health communication's multi-disciplinary reach, further study, application, and appreciation of economic, political, and other related areas should also be explored, including theories on public opinion, polling, perception and education (Price & Roberts 1987, Ratzan 1989), and other societal influences that impact health behaviors.

The development of a successful strategy for disseminating health information mandates the application and knowledge of theoretical precepts. Even with the scarcity and limitations of time, money, and environmental constraints, the strategic health communicator must still use "all the available means of persuasion" advanced by Aristotle 2000 years ago to effect an audience (see Aristotle 1984). What this calls for is an ethical perspective – the testing and questioning of assumptions of variables, the respective relationship of such variables that often define the foundation for message design. Yet, any ideal communication intervention recognizes that such strategies are a *means not an end*. Delivering the message to the intended receiver is a most important step that mandates clarification, deliberation, and feedback among individuals at many different levels in the co-ordinated effort to ultimately effect a decision.

The operative definition of *health communication* thus is: **"The process and effect of employing ethical persuasive means in human health care decision-making" (Ratzan 1993: 5).**

Theory into action

All of these theories include strategies that advance knowledge and common sense. It is the goal of the author to outline virtues for health communicators to be cognizant in their attempts to involve the essential "participants" in the process of disseminating appropriate information. Those ultimately affected by the decision – the individual on their health – represent the rubric of "humankind": they are the patient/family, the provider and society at large.

Four distinct strategies that are predominantly employed in health communication will be offered. Although most health interventions do not neatly fit into a given category, they provide a framework for analysis.

Public relations

One of the greatest leaders in the US once said: "Public Opinion is everything. With public sentiment nothing can fail; without it nothing can succeed. Consequently, he who molds public opinion goes deeper than he who enacts statutes or pronounces decisions." Although President Abraham Lincoln made this pronouncement over a hundred years ago, its relevance endures in today's global village.

An important mechanism used to disseminate health information is rooted in the field of *public relations.* The public relations professional is viewed as the principal press agent releasing information to the media. The ideal public relations agent cultivates professional and social relationships with key "publics" whose associations with the media, opinion leaders or others facilitate their client's mission of disseminating health related information. In most cases, such information is created with traditional channels of communication – newsletters, newspapers, mass media (television, radio and film) – or new technologies such as world wide web.

However, public relations is not mere press agentry. Public relations is often described as the "relating to the public" with the art of adjusting organizations to environments and environments to organizations. Public relations activities have dual rhetorical goals: interpreting the perspectives of relevant publics to members of an organization's management team, and "defining" the organization for relevant publics. The public relations emphasis is on promoting an *organization*, rather than advancing its *product.*

The public relations practitioner's goal is to build support for an organization or cause, to enhance its credibility, and/or to manage the predictable and unforeseen crises that may affect the organization's ability to meet its objectives. For a successful public relations encounter, a strong ethical component/bond ought to exist between the client and agent. The client and agent should know and have mutually agreed upon the goals of the relationship. In theory, and hopefully in practice, each plays a synergistic role in the public relations encounter.

Public relations is an obvious strategic mode to effective health communication messages. Frequently, public health groups engage in public relations efforts without the actual knowledge they are engaging in such activity. Yet, in today's world of special events marketing and political and cause campaigns, the public relations practitioner is not the sole owner of press releases, "generated" media coverage, advertisements, and sponsored events.

Public relations efforts are principally aimed toward building *strategic relationships* – a process that is facilitated by establishing an image of high ethos, formative research, audience segmentation, and channel selection, characteristics that are also employed in other approaches to health communication to be described later (Winett and Wallack 1996).

Negotiation

Health communication in a negotiation framework places the ethical responsibility on both the sender and receiver to participate actively in finding common participating responses to a shared exigence (Bitzer 1968). In the "health situation", the exigence requires an appropriate response – whether it be reassurance, restrictions, aggressive intervention(s) or the gathering of information. Health communication is commonly examined as requiring shared decision making; a negotiation perspective also subsumes such grounding.

A proactive negotiation approach has the potential to significantly affect various levels of health and to contribute to an informed citizenry. Furthermore, a negotiation perspective can improve the quality and the delivery of health care, as well as broaden the attitudes and beliefs of healthcare providers and consumers.

Advances in the art of negotiation and its prudent use of concepts from decision science and mathematics (i.e. probability) are concomitant with the revolutionary changes in medicine. However, even with precise measurement techniques at our disposal, it is impossible to derive a reliable quantitative instrument capable and reliable for effective health decision making. An example of shared decision-making success is a workable integrative negotiation (WIN) approach. Although published and applied in a variety of contexts (for examples see Kroger 1994; Ratzan 1993a,b; 1994; 1995; 1996; Ratzan et al. 1994) an abridged general explanation of WIN is presented here which will serve as a foundation for its subsequent application in health communication. WIN advances a variety of communication principles and employs a hypothetico-deductive model (Campbell 1987). The WIN approach is based in communication; accordingly shared decision-making begins and ends with the art of communication.

As a negotiation process, WIN follows a simple acronym – COAST (Communication, Options, Alternatives, Standards, Trust, see Ch. 9). COAST originates with the initial communication act between individuals or players, which includes sharing and defining interests, establishing agendas with appropriate attention to constraints of time and place, as well as listening and identifying cultural variables including verbal and nonverbal behavior. As this joint decision-making process further matures, all involved parties are invited to present options through brainstorming (without judgment), and then to deduce and to prioritize, as appropriate, acceptable alternatives.

This important negotiation act occurs with an understanding of mutually agreed upon objective standards. Open participatory integrative negotiation imbues the process with trust, a synergistic, welcomed side effect. The ultimate result is a satisfactory and successful outcome. The product of a most important foundation – an effective ongoing relationship.

In the absence of a context permeated by trust, any decision rendered is transitory at best. Once parties agree upon a decision with workable integrative negotiation, the trust inherent within the process translates into what negotiation terminology defines as "a compliance-prone agreement" (e.g. "I will not eat beef that has been potentially fed other animal sources that might have infectious agents, based on health grounds"). Given the dynamic and ongoing nature of this process, the COAST model empowers individuals to continue a strategic approach to decision making about health issues. This completes the initial cycle; the result – a relationship in the health situation.

The underlying premise of negotiation is as follows: the benefit of mutually satisfying and trusting relationships with potential stakeholders, opinion leaders, gatekeepers, allies, and the community-at-large, empowered decision-makers (consumers, clients or leaders) to make the best decision.

The COAST workable integrative negotiation process suggests an active participation by the individual or his/her designate in implementing self determinism to effect his/her overall health and well-being. The process builds upon the reciprocal respect and credibility of its constituents, employing various means and modes of information exchange, each dependent upon the context, the audience and the objective. The abiding ethical goal is to enhance trust while advocating and implementing specific actions to improve the public good. Such an idea of enhancing partnerships is an essential part of negotiation, especially in dealing with risk.

The negotiation approach is centered in active participation; the crucial constituent in effective healthcare decision making is the individual patient,[1] the root of the locus of control for the ultimate decision of their own (and society's at large) health. The defining characteristic in WIN is that two or more people participate and address the health exigence.

Negotiation ultimately establishes agreed upon agendas consistent with the interests, needs, rules, norms and concerns of the appropriate parties involved in the decision making in the health situation.

Advocacy

In 1854, when 500 people died of cholera in ten days, Dr John Snow uncovered the epidemiological reason – all lived within 250 yards of the same water pump. When Dr Snow intervened by engineering the removal of the handle of the water pump, the epidemic ended in three days. People were protected – not because of an individual behavior change – but due to a change in the environment.

Practitioners of advocacy approach public health issues from a systemic level by primarily focusing on those factors in the social, economic, and political environments that predispose populations to poor health. The goal is simple: change the systemic variables that adversely affect health status. Ultimately, the advocacy approach generally involves mobilization of the media. As such it combines community organizing strategies with the power of the mass media in the consolidated effort to influence powerholders to advance specific health-promoting policy initiatives. Such an approach is generally termed media advocacy with its use of media resources to advocate a cause (Winett & Wallack 1996). Advocacy in the formulation and coalitions of groups and organizations in building social movements (Weick 1979, Fabj & Sobnosky 1993) is termed social advocacy.

Media advocacy addresses the system-level variables that are implicated in the perpetuation of poor health (United States Department of Health and Human Services 1988, Wallack 1990). While the previously discussed communication orientations addressed issues of *information* and *behavior* in reducing disease, media advocacy strives to address the gaps in *power* and *resources* that are predictive of poor health (Wallack et al. 1993).

Media advocacy has been defined as "the strategic use of mass media as a resource for advancing a social or public policy initiative" (United States Department of Health and Human Services 1988). It is a component of comprehensive advocacy efforts designed to facilitate community-level groups ability to influence public debate by: (1) putting pressure on policymakers; (2) increasing the volume of the public health voice; and, in turn (3) increasing the visibility of values, people, and issues behind the voice (Wallack et al. 1993).

This strategy is about more than just "getting press". It is about studying and influencing how an issue is presented in the media, placing issues on the political/public agenda, and moving the debate about public policy to social causes and solutions.

While the primary target of media advocacy is to exert pressure on those with the power to make health-promoting policy-level changes in the social environment, it also attempts to reach other opinion leaders and funders, as well as other potential advocates of the general public. From a strategy perspective, media advocacy – like public relations – involves the use of paid and earned media to accomplish its goals. The hopeful outcome of the advocate is to (1), set the policy agenda, (2) shape the debate and/or (3) advance the policy.

To the novice, media advocacy and public relations strategies may appear similar. The content of media advocacy-based messages is on advancing policy goals. Attention is focused away from the "individual responsibility" to the public orientation, also favored in public relations, negotiation, and social marketing. Yet, media coverage earned for public relations efforts is not so predisposed. Media advocacy-generated news coverage characteristically strives to reframe health problems from individual matters to public issues. The public issue is transformed from a problem of *individual responsibility* to the best interest of *all in society*. It allows government and policy-makers to employ a substituted judgment of how society ought to act (e.g. one should not litter to keep the environment clean, driving drunk is not acceptable, etc.) rather than relying on the individual decision to act appropriately.

Supporters argue that media advocacy should be used as a component, among others, in an integrated effort to promote public health; comprehensive solutions to public health problems should ideally address the multiple sources of poor health in populations, both at individual and socio-systemic levels (Wallack 1990, Wallack et al. 1993). Because most discussion of health status occurs at the individual level, media advocacy strives to extend public debate to include those systemic factors that other strategies tend to bypass on what becomes an increasingly completed road to a healthier society.

Additionally, the controversy-generated "attention" that may often result from media advocacy initiatives is viewed by its proponents as precisely the needed element to effect widespread changes in public health status.

Social marketing

The Centers for Disease Control and Prevention (CDC) has derived a social marketing perspective in its approach to health communication: "the crafting and delivery of messages and strategies, based on consumer research, to promote the health of individuals and communities" (CDC 1991).

The basis of modern day social marketing principles is rooted in the Hippocratic and Greek rhetorical teaching of knowing one's audience. The writings of Hippocrates offer prescriptive ideas on the best means to render diagnosis and treatment: "[One must learn] from the common nature of all and the particular nature of the individual, from the disease, the patient, the regimen prescribed and the prescriber – for these make a diagnosis more favorable or less; from the constitution, both as a whole and with respect to the parts, of the weather and of the region; from the custom, mode of life, practices and ages of each patient; from talk, manner, silence, thoughts, sleep, absence of sleep, the nature and time of dreams, pluckings, scratching, tears ..." [Hippocrates 1984: Epidemics XXIII, 181].

Social marketing involves the integration of marketing principles and social psychology in the comprehensive efforts to "market" socially beneficial ideas, behaviors, or beliefs to targeted populations (Lefebvre & Flora 1988, Kotler & Roberto 1989, Walsh et al. 1993).

Social marketing is defined as "a social-change management technology involving the design, implementation, and control of programs aimed at increasing the acceptability of a social idea or practice in one or more groups of target adopters" (Kotler & Roberto 1989: 24).

Social marketing is a term used for the application of marketing practices to nonprofit and social purposes (Ling et al. 1992). There are several distinctions between "social marketing" and "commercial marketing". Marketing professionals in the business domain generally sell tangible products that offer near-instant gratification in exchange for financial compensation. Social marketers often promote intangible, delayed or probabilistic health benefits that frequently involve consumers expending time and energy to learn new skills, or making difficult changes in their lifestyle habits.

The principal objective of social marketing is to change the behavior of a target audience by (1) minimizing the barriers to acceptance of the costs, and (2) maximizing the potential benefits for adoption of the innovation/intervention. In the traditional application of social marketing, the goal is to impart knowledge, generate emotion, garner support, model skills, and stimulate information-seeking within audiences; the focus is on the *channel and audience*. Appropriate appeals are crafted with research and testing and subsequently delivered in order to persuade audiences to voluntarily adopt the new health "product" – information, ideas, or behaviors – for some "exchange" of commitment, time, money, and/or physical/mental energy or a restructure of personal belief systems. Fred Kroger of the CDC, originator of numerous health communication strategies, also reminds us of the importance of creativity in designing an appropriate appeal in social marketing: "The solution may call for health communicators to place as much of their scientific and creative energizes on issues of distribution as they do on message design and packaging" (CDC 1991).

The most widely used social marketing strategy in health communication is segmentation, partitioning a total audience into sub-audiences that are each relatively homogeneous in the segmentation variable (for example, risk factors like IV drug use for HIV/AIDS prevention). More effective health messages are created for each audience partition or segment rather than for the entire audience.

Social marketing is characterized by its strong emphasis on the needs and preferences of target audiences given that successful persuasion application would include the audience's involvement with the topic, recognition and knowledge of the problem, past experience, expectations, social norms, time availability, use of language, and values. Research suggests that members of the target audience must be involved in developing message strategies, at least in terms of providing formative input (Maibach et al. 1993, Palmer 1981).

In contrast to negotiation or advocacy, social marketing is described as a "responsive" process of communication that *originates* with the public health organization, not the audience; its message reflects the expressed and identified preferences of the target audience (Walsh et al. 1993). However, true participatory planning is complicated by geographically diverse target audiences, by large social distances between campaign planners and target audiences, and by bureaucratic factors that inhibit the involvement of audience members.

Discussion

The Greek physician Herophilus observed over 2000 years ago that illness renders science null, art inglorious, strength effortless, wealth useless, and eloquence powerless (Owen 1996). The mad cow exigence did much the same to the body politic. An appropriate strategic communication strategy either individually or as a hybrid can assist those who deliver health. Just as in disease, it is easier to prevent rather than cure the ills of conflict.

An underlying principle in all of the health communication strategies discussed is that the health communicator has an ethical responsibility to act appropriately. The purpose of this chapter is not an elucidation of the ethical dilemmas in opting for one strategy over another. Yet, the ideals of deontologic ethics – (i.e. right and wrong is clear with a duty to obey absolute principles) and teleologic ethics (i.e. judge the ethicality of actions according to consequences and the level of greatest good for the greatest number of people) – ought to be considered in the decision-making process. The health communicator's decision to choose a mode of action is often determined only in the particular training of the individual or in the solutions often offered by culture and society.

For example, the social marketing perspective follows the best interest of the community at large – (i.e. one making the best decision for many), while the negotiation perspective focuses on the individual's autonomy and decision-making ability (i.e. involving the audience to determine the decision best for him/her). From a philosophical perspective, social marketing has been criticized for promoting single solutions to complex health problems while often ignoring the environmental precursors that might cause and/or sustain disease (Wallack 1990). Media advocacy and public relations often are limited in their scope to address issues that solely affect a vocal or well-funded group in society rather than the organized whole. However, applied together such strategies can be successful.

According to Backer et al. (1992), effective health communication combines mass media with organizational, community, and interpersonal activities, comprising a so-called "systems" approach to communication campaigns. Furthermore, conventional wisdom suggests that mechanisms that facilitate accurate face-to-face channels of communication are more effective, and essential in inducing ultimate behavior change. Table 15.1 summarizes such approaches.

Guidelines

The following questions provide a framework for anyone involved in the dissemination of health information. Just as research design and the actual scientific study require a certain wherewithal of time, energy and resources, strategic decision making and research is of equal importance prior to implementing a course of action:

A dozen questions for a health communicator to answer while choosing an orientation to influence public health

(1) Define the health problem. Identify the reasons/explanation – who, what, where, when, why, how and how many (magnitude)?

Table 15.1 Comparison of the fundamental characteristics of four orientations (organization and certain orientations reprinted from Winett and Wallack 1996).

Approach	Social marketing	Public relations	Advocacy	Negotiation
Source of action	Agency or organization	Agency or organization	Community or collaborative	Individual or community agency or organization
Focus	develops health messages to increase knowledge and model behaviors; enhances image of sponsoring organization	develops messages and cultivates relationships in order to enhance the organization's associations with key publics	<ul><li>setting the agenda</li><li>shaping the debate</li><li>advancing the policy</li><li>policies enacted to improve health</li></ul>	<ul><li>determining the agenda</li><li>building coalitions</li><li>influencing the policy</li><li>compliance-prone decisions to improve health</li></ul>
Target of media efforts	<ul><li>individuals with risk factors</li><li>general public</li></ul>	<ul><li>customers, clients, shareholders, and current funders</li><li>potential supporters and funders</li><li>general public</li></ul>	<ul><li>power holders and policy makers</li><li>producers, marketers of health-affecting products</li><li>other advocates</li><li>general public</li></ul>	<ul><li>stakeholders and decision-makers</li><li>professionals, producers, marketers of health-affecting products and services</li><li>social networks</li><li>general public – individuals</li></ul>
Perceived need to be filled by media strategy	knowledge and behavior deficit	knowledge and familiarity deficit	power and resource deficit	knowledge, power and participatory behavior deficit

Method	Create an optimum blend of the 4P's of marketing in order to reduce the target audience's perceived barriers to accepting the product, while simultaneously making the product as appealing as possible May utilize free or paid media	Cultivate relationships, project desired image, and maintain visible community involvement in order to promote "favorable associations" with key publics Use "earned" news media and paid advertising to gain exposure for organization	Utilize "earned" news media and paid advertising, in conjunction with community organization strategies, to put pressure on policy makers and to reframe public debate on an issue	Identify decision-makers at all levels that can influence and be involved with helping the individuals to render their own decisions and build trusting relationships for future benefit Promotes a healthy citizen responsible for her/his own actions
Mode of action	can be used in isolation, or as part of larger efforts	can be used alone, or as part of integrated communications efforts	used in combination with other community organization and advocacy strategies	can be used alone, or as part of integrated communication efforts with community organization and advocacy strategies
Level of effect	Primarily individual	Primarily individual	Primarily social environment	Individual to social environment and policy-makers

(2) Is there a need to respond to the problem (e.g. scientific report, news, etc.)?

(3) Are the causes of the problem readily identifiable? If so, could you effectively and efficiently address the problem?

(4) Is the health problem one that should be addressed through the public receiving information, modeling behavior or gathering recommendations?

(5) Is the health problem one that can be solved through identifying short-term behavior changes to specific audiences (e.g. wash utensils, boil water, don't eat cheese from a certain producer)?

(6) Is the problem one that could be addressed by choosing a sender with increased credibility (e.g. surgeon general)?

(7) Is the problem one requiring education and collaboration with other organizations, opinion leaders, clients, powerholders, or the general public?

(8) Is the problem widespread and capable of being solved through individual, community, workplace, or governmental action?

(9) Are there multiple parties effected by the problem in different ways (e.g. harms, benefits, advantages and disadvantages, etc.)?

(10) What are the desired outcomes of the communication intervention? How do these relate to the overall health objectives?

(11) Will media strategies be central or peripheral to the health campaign?

(12) What kind of resources are available, including money, time, equipment, expertise, creativity, and person-power?

Approach

The following section presents individual strategies based on the previously mentioned theories that might have been employed to address such a crisis and limit its escalation.

Each of the approaches discussed earlier offers different merits and limitations, depending upon the *context* of a given public health issue and the overall interests of the individual/organization working to affect it. It should be obvious to the practitioner that none of the approaches is mutually exclusive. There is a functional overlap for health communication experts. The most comprehensive approach for public health professionals is one that blends such strategies with a common ethical underpinning.

Social Marketing

The basic premise of social marketing is that when presented with the optimal blend of behavioral, interpersonal, and environmental cues, target audiences can be persuaded to accept the product, behavior, value, idea or belief being promoted (Kotler & Roberto 1989, Walsh et al. 1993). This health communication intervention occurs through an ideal mix of marketing's "four P's" – product, price, place and promotion. A chart applied to the mad cow case is provided in Table 15.2.

A social marketing perspective affords opportunities to educate, increase support for an issue, and promote short-term changes in health behaviors. Social marketers could craft messages that both acknowledge and directly address the preferences of specific audiences in order to present the most persuasive arguments targeting individual risk factors. Social marketing could effect change at the individual level. In this case, a strategy could encompass a public relations approach. There could have been appropriate preparation used *prior* to the 1996 exigence that evolved into the major crisis. For years there was discussion and debate on the potential link between mad cow disease and CJD and the related areas of questions of safety. If the public had understood that there were no infectious agents ever found in the beef for human consumption (prions have never been isolated in muscle) or in any beef products, they would not have reacted in such a swift manner by avoiding products that did not have any potential for transmission of disease.

Given the widespread cultural value and habit in the UK and in Europe with beef consumption, the availability and accessibility of beef products, and the nutritional value and the positive effects people often experience while choosing beef over other food products – the social marketing perspective could have played a significant role in addressing the issue, i.e. that the benefits outweigh the overstated potential infinitesimal risk. In this instance, social marketers would have to "sell" the fact there is *no link* to disease and reaffirm the scientific uncertainty and overstated claim. While the likelihood of a social marketing campaign succeeding solely using the "beef is good and safe" campaign would be minimal, it nonetheless could advance dialogue on the weak association of death in a limited number of cases that might be due to ingestion of beef or beef products.

Social marketers could use multiple channels to disseminate the message. The use of paid advertisements on television, radio and in print, creation of fact lines (i.e. web sites, hotlines and other such venues), point of purchase (i.e. butcher shops) for factual information and other such areas should have been mobilized immediately. The marketing strategies to disseminate information on beef could include millions of intermediaries in the form of grocers, druggists, truck drivers, packagers, restaurateurs, farmers, and the like, few of whom are trained in health communication *per se*, but all of whom willingly participate in a strategically designed marketing system to accurately inform the public. Further, mechanisms to educate the policy-makers, such as the use of cassette tapes in different languages with concise messages of the scientific facts, could have been developed and disseminated. Instead, the repetitive messages were derived by the media interested in conflict and sensationalism over facts.

Table 15.2 The four P's of social marketing

Element	Definition	Ideal approach: British beef is safe to eat
Product	What, in terms of attitude, behavior, beliefs, information, or services, is the audience being asked to accept	Ideal message: There is no risk of getting CJD by eating British beef: • target audiences learning about CJD as a rare brain disease NOT definitively linked to mad cow disease • target audiences restoring faith maintain safe beef-eating habits • community-wide increases in the availability of information about beef safety in cafeterias, restaurants and purchase points • information that the infectious agent of mad cow disease has never been found in red meat
Price	The cost – financial, social, material, physical, and/or psychological – that the target audience is being asked to voluntarily contribute in exchange for accepting the product	Target audiences experience: • consumers switch to other products • farmers loss of livelihood • necessity to change farming practice of offal feed • grocers/butchers decreased sales • loss of market share of the $4 billion industry • restaurants decrease in sales and increased effort and costs associated with cultivating new menus and patrons • customers protesting unsafe products • policymakers rushing to judgment to eliminate beef for public consumption • international outcry to protect markets and citizens • uncertainty of scientific discovery on health issues
Place	The distribution channels dictating how and where the product will be made available to the target audience for trial and/or for acceptance. This variable refers to both the physical availability	• broadcasting and/or publishing educational and skills-building components of the newspapers, on television, and radio stations frequented by target audience members and their supporters • providing mad cow updates and health information ensuring

	and the social availability of the product being marketed from the perspectives of target audience members	"healthy" disease-free beef in local grocery stores and restaurants • providing opinion leaders, role models and educators at community events and social centers • motivating support systems by enjoining opinion leaders and soliciting the involvement of organizations at both the scientific and local community levels • providing target audiences with opportunities to ask questions get information and get feedback/answers • providing follow-up opportunities with credible sources – educators and government officials/appointees to reinforce consumer confidence • providing support and resources to point of purchase/point of consumption areas – markets, restaurants and cafeterias
Promotion	How the target audience will be made aware of the product and its availability, and how this awareness will be translated into audience members' intention to accept the product	Engaging a variety of mass media and interpersonal channels to: • provide credible sources to describe the current state of knowledge about the mad cow linkage to feed, sheep, veal and humans • provide credible members to advocate for and demonstrate the merits of the information that beef will not cause human death • providing immediate incentives for compliance and rewards for meeting goals by reporting mad cow and keeping it our of the food supply • mobilizing widespread social support systems for the desired behaviors; engaging broad organization and community involvement in campaign activities • providing ongoing opportunities for new information dissemination with credible sources

Public Relations

Table 15.3 offers some generic assistance in a public relations approach with emphasis on the media strategy.

Public relations strategies offer a means to promote an organization and its image, to build strategic relationships, and to cultivate supportive social

Table 15.3 A public relations approach

Public relations	
Source of action	Agency or organization
Proactive	Study the patterns and type of reporting in your target area and determine which media representative (tv, print, radio, etc) are the most effective and knowledgeable. Contact each to develop and cultivate relationships in order to enhance the organization's associations with key publics Formulate alliances with other representatives of similar interest(s)
Strategy	Be able to write and articulate a strategy not just with facts but with messages and images
Long-term societal goals of agency	Continue to advance the importance of your organization and relate it to the overall role of the health of the public
Image	Maintain a high integrity image of truthfulness, expertise and candor while cultivating relationships, and maintaining visible community involvement in order to promote "favorable associations" with key publics Use "earned" news media and paid advertising to gain exposure for organization. Redistribute such information in press kits, newsletters and other image enhancing vehicles
Crisis interaction	Always be responsive to queries, whether directly related to your primary issue. The media representatives remember who helped them
Individual goal	Trustworthy information and strategic relationships

climates. Public relations generally enhances the opportunity to access key publics and avoid problems in an attempt to positively affect factors in social, institutional, and political environments. In this case there was no clear public relations strategy, only the hastily determined release of the SEAC report by the British Government. The initial announcement lacked a plan to choose a primary spokesperson who would be the credible "voice". Additionally, the failure to act quickly after the initial announcement to provide the facts and the implications of those facts in a credible manner, fueled speculation and hearsay. Public relations efforts could have elicited relationships with key media, the McDonalds corporation, policy-makers and related groups, to create a crisis communication team and an expert group to avert a crisis. However, with over ten years of purported public relations efforts, there were insufficient relationships to disseminate information with a common voice. The fact there was no clear agency or voice was a major blunder. Hence the decision by McDonalds to eliminate British beef became the actual policy all would follow. The UK Government lost control of the agenda as they were out of touch with certain organizations and let the market place drive policy. Appropriate advocacy to restore consumer confidence could have focused on safety over elimination of the "menace".

Negotiation

For a WIN strategy of negotiation, see Table 15.4.

When health communication involves a message of communication of risk, a negotiation approach is a most important strategy. The National Research Council (1996) report reminds readers of the importance of understanding risk communication as "... an interactive process of exchange of information, and opinion among individuals, groups and institutions. It involves multiple messages about the nature of risk and other messages, not strictly about risk, that express concerns, opinions or reactions to risk messages or to legal and institutional arrangements for risk management." Hence, risk communication commands what Maibach & Holgrave (1995: 223) term "truly interactive communication and shared decision-making about risk-management strategies." In the case of the beef crisis, the apt health communicator would embody these ideals with a negotiation approach. For example, with the identification of the stakeholders in society – from the consumer to the butcher to the farmer to the health official to the policymaker – each could work on similar interests to have a safe source of food. A representative approach of the COAST model is in Table 15.4. Although it is presented in a static format, it could have evolved with the different players focusing on the appropriate venues. The negotation approach affords an opportunity to select the optimal components from the other strategies. Ideally, participants "buy in" to the decision and enhance the potential for its success. However, given the complexity of the issue, it is important that the chosen

Table 15.4 Workable integrative negotiation strategy of communication

	Consumer - Public	Government - UK	Europeans	Media
Communication	Safety of food supply Purchase power and information Need for accurate and factual information	Protection of citizens/industry Own safeguards regarding domestic regulations Competing agendas for market share	Safety and Autonomy European Union and sovereignty of nations in decisions Not British but European problem	Information for the public Maintain interest in the issue Portray conflicting ideas, roles and responsibilities
Options	• stop buying beef • get accurate info • find answers on government hot-line number	• regulate beef • develop a test for BSE • restore consumer confidence • "fight" the European Union and defy	• regulate British products – ban beef or all trade • maintain leadership and power • protect member states	• determine the cause • maintain interest • establish credibility • serve as resource for information • bring science in the debate
Alternatives	• best alternative – switch to other meats • wait for the answer	• restore confidence • maintain control • protect market • block legislation	• protect European health and economy • maintain agricultural policymaking • protect market	• publish all findings as they are released • advance the issue with human interest • keep conflict as focus
Standards	• "they say" – leaders and scientists	• data from scientists	• past legislation; precedents of legislation/policy making • power to enforce blockade	• information from any source that is "new" is news

Trust	Create power as concerned consumers, farmers, citizens, scientists etc. Try to identify mechanism for information from reliable sources	Develop relationships and power structures with all concerned parties – farmers, consumers, meat processors, regulators etc. Create individual/group/body as consistent spokesperson. Build ethos through message consistency	Forge agreements that protect each interested party. Allow individual concerns raised in private, but keep all actions of solidarity in public. Establish communication with UK and media with consistent message.	Continue to get individuals to advance their own agenda in public to spur controversy Advance stereotypes through highlighting German embargo. Consider Europhiles/phobes, yes/no, black/white un/certainty issues with explanations and headlines
Suggested action	Demand accurate information from all sources over a variety of channels	Continue to advance the message/theme: No risk to humans ever proven – infectious agent never found in cow meat	Hold EU together by negotiating behind closed doors with a plan to eradicate BSE and restore confidence. Act swiftly and in agreement for a majority vote	Act in responsible way as public educator. Rather than spur speculation, advance the dialogue and examine the facts
Actual effectiveness	Weakest player individually; must organize and advocate	Reactive rather than proactive	Havoc, derailment of actions, lack of confidence in government	Continued cynicism in government and media reports

negotiators be extremely competent to involve each party successfully in the process.

Advocacy

Advocacy could have been used to help change the environment so that individuals could make healthy and realistic choices based on trustworthy information. The media could have been used as effective channels in the largest venue by emphasizing public health from a "public" perspective. An advocacy approach is outlined in Table 15.5 and focuses on changing the environment in which people act, hopefully enhancing their ease to make the best decisions for the largest number of people. It can be more successful in a speedy fashion as it could influence the system rather than relying on an individual to make all of the decisions solely from a "personal" perspective.

In this case an amalgam of the strengths and potentials of each strategy is paramount. In the beef crisis, organization for a swift and speedy response from the farming industry, consumer coalitions, beef retailers and others at the grassroots level with appropriate supporting data could have helped frame the issue as a government mistake, rather than an issue of consumer confidence. Given the multiple levels of involvement in this case, a pan-Europe approach would be most effective, targeted at decision-makers in key regions.

Conclusion

Using the criteria described here, a leader, communication professional or strategist can apply their knowledge and experience to the issue – in combination with the causes of, and best ways to address, poor health. The optimum professional would select from the characteristics, capabilities, and limitations of the four communication orientations briefly outlined in this chapter.

Although scientists are aware that scientific progress is anachronistic, nearly three-quarters of the public is skeptical about the accuracy of the news. While the public is cynical of the factual nature of material, all of us are forced to digest information instantaneously from limited sources, making decisions without the opportunity to discriminate among values and weigh the evidence. We have limited guidance from our once trusted physician, now reduced to a healthcare provider. What is necessary is a strategic approach – an amalgam of public relations, social marketing, negotiation and advocacy from credible sources to truly inform the public. However, if finite resources are of concern, an organization may need to restrict its choice of strategies to those with the greatest potential for achieving its objective of dissemination of accurate information.

Such issues present important challenges in a society where perception has become *de facto* reality. With the current societal void in promoting

Table 15.5 An advocacy approach

Advocacy	
Source of action	Community or collaborative or media.
Proactive	Defining and framing of the issue in a macro-context to attract support of credible sources. Cattleman's, farmers and other unions educating key publics on their role. Integrating scientists in the "team".
Strategy	Become an active "player" in the dissemination of information. Mobilize key groups to "create" news by presenting the issues to the general public through social organization (i.e. march on Downing Street) and media mobilization.
Long-term societal goals of agency	Get on the radar screen with full scale political campaign against those with differing interests. Mobilize those with similar interests.
Method/Image	Create an issue with regard to the ultimate goal – to put pressure on policy makers and to make a decision on behalf of your interests. Utilize the news media and paid advertising, in conjunction with community organization strategies.
Intervention	Be able to mobilize the organization immediately with new technologies, fax, e-mail etc. to raise the issue and be a presence as soon as possible.
Individual Goal	Change the environment.

accurate health knowledge, those involved in the discovery and dissemination of health-related information should also be involved in dissemination of their findings. They must have dual roles as ethical educators presenting objective and accurate health information. Advocating such an outlook, all of us should work to protect, maintain and advance our most vital asset – health.

Notes

Special acknowledgement: The author would like to add special thanks and reference Winett L. & L. Wallack (1996) "Advancing public health goals through the mass media", *Journal of Health Communication*, **1**(2) 173–96, 1996.

1 The word client is chosen here although we would add another acronym to this chapter. A "PATIENT" is a Person Advocating Their Interests Effectively Negotiating Treatment.

References

Aristotle 1984. *Rhetoric*. London: William Heinemann.

Ajzen, I. & M. Fishbein 1980. *Understanding attitudes and predicting social behavior*. Englewood Cliffs, New Jersey: Prentice Hall.

Backer T., E. Rogers & P. Sopory 1992. *Designing health communication campaigns: what works?* Newbury Park: Sage.

Bandura, A. 1986. *Social foundations of thought and action: A social cognitive approach*. Englewood Cliffs, New Jersey: Prentice Hall.

Bitzer, L. 1968. The rhetorical situation. *Philosophy and Rhetoric* **1**, 1–6.

Campbell, E. J. M. 1987. The diagnosing mind. *Lancet* **1**, 849–51.

Centers for Disease Control and Prevention 1991. Health communications at the Centers for Disease Control: current status and recommendations. July, Atlanta, Georgia.

Dearing, J. W. & E. M. Rogers 1996. *Agenda-setting*. Newbury Park: Sage.

Fabj, V. & M. J. Sobnosky 1993. Responses from the Street: ACT UP and Community Organizing against AIDS. In *AIDS: effective health communication for the 90's* 91–109 S. C. Ratzan, (ed.). Washington, DC: Taylor & Francis.

Fisher, R. & W. Ury 1981. *Getting to yes*. New York: Penguin.

Hippocrates 1984. *Hippocrates*. London: Heinemann.

Janis, I.L. & S. Feshbach 1953. Effects of fear arousing communications. *Journal of Abnormal and Social Psychology* **48**, 78–92

Kahneman, D. & A. Tversky 1972. Subjective probability: a judgement of representativeness. *Cognitive Psychology* **3**, 430–54.

Kotler, P. & E. L. Roberto 1989. *Social marketing: strategies for changing public behavior*. New York: The Free Press.

Kroger, F. 1994. Toward a healthy public. *American Behavioral Scientist* **38**(2), 215–23.

Lasswell, H. D. 1972. Communication research and public policy, *Public Opinion Quarterly* **36**, 301–10.

Lefebvre, R. C. & J. Flora 1988. Social marketing and public health intervention. *Health Education Quarterly* **15**(3), 299–315.

Ling, J. C., B. A. K. Franklin, J. F. Lindsteadt, S. A. N. Gearon 1992. Social marketing: its place in public health. *Annual Review of Public Health* **13**, 341–62.

Maibach, E. M., G. L. Kreps, E. W. Bonaguro 1993. Developing strategic communication campaigns for HIV/AIDS prevention. In *AIDS: effective health communication for the 90's* S. C. Ratzan (ed.). Washington: Taylor & Francis.

Maibach, E. M. & Holtgrave 1995. Advances in public health communication. *Annual Review of Public Health* **16**, 219–38.

McCombs, M. & D. Shaw 1972. The agenda setting function of the mass media. *Public Opinion Quarterly* **36**, 176–87.

McGuire, W. J. 1989. Theoretical foundations of campaigns. In *Public Communication Campaigns*, 2nd edn R. Rice & C. Atkin (eds). 43–67. Newbury Park: Sage.

National Research Council 1989. *Improving Risk Communication*. Committee on Risk Perception and Communication. Washington DC: National Academy Press.

Owen, L. D. 1996. A clinician's caution, rhetoric and reality. In *Preventive Diplomacy* K. Cahill (ed.) Basic Books.

Palmer, E. 1981. Shaping persuasive messages with formative research. In *Public Communication Campaigns*, 2nd edn. R. Rice & C. Atkin (eds). Newbury Park: Sage.

Payne, J. G., S. C. Ratzan, R. A. Baukus 1989. Dissemination of news in the Harvard Medicare Project: regional/discreet differences. *Health Communication* **1**(4), 220–45.

Price, V. & D. Roberts 1987. Public opinion processes. In *Handbook of communication science* C. Berger & S. Chafee (eds). Newbury Park: Sage.

Ratzan, S. 1989. The real agenda setters. *American Behavioral Scientist* **32**(4), 451–63.

Ratzan, S. C. 1993a. Health communication and AIDS; setting the agenda. In *AIDS: effective health communication for the 90's* Ratzan, S. C. (ed.). Washington: Taylor & Francis.

Ratzan, S. C. 1993b. Political communication as negotiation. *American Behavioral Scientist* **37**, 200–10.

Ratzan, S. C. 1994. The healthy American act. *American Behavioral Scientist* **38**, 224–7.

Ratzan, S. C. 1995. Ethical decision making in managing trauma. *Neurosurgery Clinics of North America* **6**(4) October.

Ratzan, S. C. 1996. Effective decision-making: a negotiation strategy for health communication and health psychology. *Journal of Health Psychology*. Newbury Park: Sage.

Ratzan, S. C., J. G. Payne and H. A. Massett 1994. Effective health message design: America responds to the AIDS campaign. *American Behavioral Scientist* **38**, 297–309.

Rogers, E. M. 1983. *Diffusion of innovations*. New York: Free Press.

Rogers, E. M. & D. Kincaid 1981. *Communication networks: toward a new paradigm for research.* New York: Free Press.

Shannon, C. E. & W. Weaver 1949. *The mathematical theory of communication.* Urbana, Illinois: University of Illinois Press.

US Department of Health and Human Services 1988. *Media strategies for smoking control guidelines.* Washington: US Department of Health and Human Services.

US Department of Health and Human Services 1991. *Healthy people 2000: national health promotion and disease prevention principles.* DHS Publications No. 91-50213. Washington: Public Health Service.

Wallack, L. 1990. Two approaches to health promotion in the mass media. *World Health Forum* **11**: 143–54.

Wallack, L., L. Dorfman, D. Jernigan, M. Themba 1993. *Media advocacy and public health: power for prevention.* Newbury Park: Sage.

Walsh, D. C., R. E. Rudd, R. A. Moeykens, T. W. Moloney 1993. Social marketing for public health. *Health Affairs* **12**(2), 104–19.

Winett L. & L. Wallack 1996. Advancing public health goals through the mass media. *Journal of Health Communication* **1**(2), 173–96.

Weick, K. 1979. *The social psychology of organizing*, 2nd edn. Reading, Massachusetts: Addison-Wesley.

Wilkes, M. S. 1997. The public dissemination of medical research: problems and solutions. *Journal of Health Communication* **2**, 1–15.

Witte, K., K. A. Cameron, J. K. McKeon, J. Berkowitz 1996. Predicting risk behaviors: development and validation of a diagnostic scale. *Journal of Health Communication* **1**, 317–41.

Zaltman, G. & R. Duncan 1977. *Strategies for planned change.* New York: John Wiley.

Appendix 1

A Chronology of BSE and CJD Developments

1976	Dr Carleton Gadjusek awarded the Nobel Prize for his work with Kuru
1982	Dr Stanley Prusiner identifies "proteinaceous infectious particles" or "prions" as the agents that cause transmissible spongiform encephalopathies
November 1986	A newly recognized form of neurological disease appears in cattle in the United Kingdom; the disease is identified as bovine spongiform encephalopathy by Gerald A. H. Wells and John W. Wilesmith of the Central Veterinary Laboratory after a post-mortem study of an affected cow
November 1986–May 1995	Approximately 150,000 cases of BSE confirmed from approximately 33,500 herds of cattle in the UK
June 1987	Transmission studies begin; normal time for disease to develop in mice proved to be about 10 months
5 December 1987	Initial epidemiology studies completed which conclude that ruminant-derived meat and bonemeal in feed was the only viable hypothesis for cause of BSE
21 April 1988	UK Government indicates that legislation would be instated to make BSE notifiable and to ban feeding of rations that contain protein derived from ruminants
21 June 1988	Provisions of BSE Order 1988 come into effect to make BSE notifiable and to provide for isolation of BSE suspects when calving
18 July 1988	Ruminant feed ban comes into force
8 August 1988	Slaughter and compensation policy comes into effect, which provides 50% compensation for confirmed BSE cases, 100% for negative, both subject to a ceiling

October 1988	Transmission to mice reported, following intracerebral inoculation of BSE brain tissue
28 November 1988	BSE made notifiable and slaughter policy introduced in Northern Ireland
30 December 1988	Feed ban prolonged, use of milk from infected animals prohibited except to feed cow's own calf
1989	Importing of processed beef and live cattle from Britain into US is stopped
11 January 1989	Use of animal protein in ruminant feed banned in Northern Ireland
28 July 1989	European Commission bans export of cattle born before 18 July 1988 and offspring of affected or suspect animals
13 November 1989	Bovine Offal Regulations come into force in England and Wales, banning the use of specified bovine offal (SBO)
30 January 1990	SBO bans come into effect in Scotland and Northern Ireland
31 January 1990	Announcement that five antelopes have succumbed to a spongiform encephalopathy
3 February 1990	Cattle to cattle transmission following intracerebral and intravenous inoculation of BSE brain tissue and into mice via the oral route reported in *Veterinary Record*
14 February 1990	Full compensation for infected animals introduced; no surge of cases associated with this introduction
30 March 1990	Administrative ban on export of specified offal and certain glands and organs (for uses other than human consumption) to other EU member states
April 1990	Spongiform Encephalopathy Advisory Committee (SEAC) is established in the UK
1 April 1990	Disease made notifiable to the European Commission
3 April 1990	Announcement made of establishment of permanent advisory group on spongiform encephalopathies under Chairmanship of Dr David Tyrrell
11 April 1990	Humberside County council withdraws British beef from school meals
10 May 1990	Announcement of a cat with a spongiform encephalopathy

17 May 1990	Announcement that decisions about breeding from offspring of affected cows should be left to individual farmers and their veterinary advisors
12 July 1990	Tyrrell Committee reports on why no need to give official advice on breeding from offspring of BSE cases
24 September 1990	Laboratory transmission of BSE to a pig announced; Tyrrell Committee advises no implications for human health, but as precaution on animal health, will ban specified offals in all animal feed (including pet food)
25 September 1990	Ban extended on use of SBO to any animal feed; exports of such feed also effectively banned to other member states
2–5 October 1990	OIE Conference in Sofia (Bulgaria); recommendations made regarding trade, prevention, control and surveillance of BSE, the support of research and the need for further consideration on trade in live animals
15 October 1990	Order passed to introduce new record-keeping arrangement requiring cattle farmers to maintain breeding records; these and movement records to be retained for ten years
27 March 1991	First case announced in BSE offspring born after ruminant feed ban
6 November 1991	BSE Order 1991 consolidates existing BSE legislation and introduces new provisions to prevent the use of meat and bonemeal produced from SBOs as a fertilizer
1992–1993	In Britain, 900 to 1,000 cows per week contract BSE
4 March 1992	Results of further experiments on the host range of BSE announced; also that the Tyrrell Committee had considered the latest BSE research and concluded that the measures at present in place provide adequate safeguards for human and animal health
14 May 1992	EC Decision prohibits intracommunity trade in bovine embryos derived from BSE suspect or confirmed dams or dams born after 18 July 1988
14 July 1993	100,000th confirmed case of BSE in Great Britain announced in response to a parliamentary Question, as an update to the UK Progress Report to the OIE
27 June 1994	Commission decision prohibits the feeding of mammalian protein to ruminants throughout EU other than Denmark

30 June 1994	Industry voluntarily extends SBO ban
27 July 1994	Commission decides to introduce new measures on beef export; requires bone-in-beef for export to come from cattle certified not to have been on holdings where BSE has been confirmed in previous six years
2 November 1994	SBO ban on human food of calves under six months of age slaughtered for human consumption; spongiform encephalopathies made notifiable in cattle, sheep and goats
6 March 1995	Restriction on use of milk, gelatin, amino acids, dicalcium phosphate and dried plasma and other blood products from mammalian tissues in feedstuffs for ruminants
1 April 1995	Regulation put into effect which makes it a requirement to stain SBO with a solution of blue ink
15 August 1995	SBO Order enacted, which consolidates and streamlines the old rules on SBO; main changes include: tighter control on record keeping, dedicated lines for rendering plants processing SBO, a prohibition on the removal of brains and eyes so that the whole skull must be disposed of as SBO, and a prohibition on the removal of the spinal cord from the vertebral column except in slaughter-houses
May 1995	BSE reported from ten countries and areas outside the UK to date; in France, Portugal, Republic of Ireland and Switzerland, BSE occurred in native cattle; in Falkland Islands, Oman Sultanate, Germany, Canada, Italy and Denmark, cases only identified in cattle imported from the UK
14 December 1995	Government bans the use of the bovine vertebral column in the manufacture of mechanically recovered meat (MRM) and other products, and prohibits the export for human consumption of MRM made from the vertebral column
December 1995	British Agriculture Minister Douglas Hogg says, "I am absolutely certain that British beef is wholly safe"
20 March 1996	SEAC states: "On current data and in the absence of any credible alternative the most likely explanation at present is that these cases are linked to exposure to BSE before the introduction of the SBO ban." Upon advice

from SEAC, the Government announces that carcasses from cattle aged over 30 months must be deboned in specially licensed plants and that the trimmings be kept out of any food chain; also that the use of mammalian meat and bonemeal in feed for all farm animals be banned

21 March 1996	First announcement of a newly recognized variant of Creutzfeldt–Jakob disease (v-CJD) in humans; the variant affects young patients (mean age 26.3 years) and has a relatively long duration of illness (mean 14.1 months); the hypothesis is announced that v-CJD may be linked to exposure to a BSE agent
24 March 1996	McDonald's suspends use of British beef in burgers
26 March 1996	Advisors confirm that v-CJD could be linked to BSE before the offal ban
29 March 1996	New regulation announced which treats entire head as SBO
2–3 April 1996	WHO, FAO and OIE participate on consultation regarding transmissible spongiform encephalopathies; report calls for more research, and a moratorium on use of potentially infected tissues from entering any food chain
10 April 1996	The Centers for Disease Control and Prevention (CDC) in the US initiates the tracking of CJD occurrences in four states: Minnesota, California, Connecticut and Oregon
12 April 1996	The US Department of Agriculture issues a report saying that transmission of BSE to humans is virtually impossible
16 April 1996	New £550 million scheme to prevent cattle most at risk from entering food chain: all beasts over 30 months old will be bought and destroyed, the purchase to be 70% funded by the EU
18 April 1996	The Government bans meat and bonemeal from sale and use as a fertilizer on agricultural land
30 April 1996	Government announces the introduction of a voluntary plan whereby farmers can use a passport to show the age of cattle; other than cases where it can be proven that the animal is no more than two years and six months old at the time of slaughter, all cattle with more than two permanent incisors are prohibited from sale for human consumption

May 1996	MAFF reports that "if there is no significant source of infection other than feed, the measures already in place will lead to the eradication of BSE"
3 May 1996	Government announces plans for a new scheme under which cattle over the age of 30 months from herds that can be identified as low risk on the basis of strict eligibility criteria may be slaughtered for human consumption
June 1996	UK Advisory Committee on Dangerous Pathogens (ACDP) acknowledges that uncertainty remains as to whether there is a causal link between BSE and human spongiform encephalopathies
6 June 1996	Five new cases of v-CJD are announced
14 June 1996	Article in *Nature* reports findings of study in which macaque monkeys were injected with BSE; produced pathology similar to v-CJD
July 1996	The US International Food Information Council (IFIC) issues an occupational warning stating that contact with, or consumption of, the brain or spinal cord of BSE-infected animals are activities that lead to risks of contracting CJD
24 July 1996	Government announces £100 million aid plan for beef producers who were affected by the fall in prices
9 August 1996	Government announces new "Beef Assurance Scheme" which allows farmers to register herds with no known risk of BSE (i.e. grass-fed cattle) to be used for human consumption up to the age of 42 months
4 October 1996	Liechtenstein reports its first case of feline spongiform encephalopathy
16 December 1996	British Government announces a change in culling plans to include cattle that were reared with animals that have died of BSE and may have eaten infected feed; also includes cattle born to cows that died of the disease
1996	Total number of confirmed cases of v-CJD: 14. 52.5% drop in confirmed BSE cases in 1996, compared to 1995
January 1997	United States Food and Drug Administration proposes ban on use of rendered cow, sheep, goat, deer and elk tissue in animal feed

2 January 1997	An article in *Nature* reports that BSE cost the EU $2.8 billion in subsidies to the beef industry
15 January 1997	30,000 tons of hamburgers, sausages, pies and lasagnes are buried in British landfill sites.
30 January 1997	UK Government announces decision to appoint a Food Safety Advisor, who will coordinate the work of existing committees and advise on the safety, quality and labeling procedures
22 February 1997	A coalition of consumer groups, veterinarians and Federal meat inspectors asks the US Government to improve the meat inspection system and to include hogs in the list of banned tissues mentioned in the proposed FDA rule
March 1997	WHO announces that three groups of people at risk for CJD should be barred from donating blood. These include recipients of growth hormones in the 1980s, recipients of dura mater, and members of families with known CJD occurrences
25 March 1997	One case of BSE diagnosed in the Netherlands in a herd that did not import cattle from known BSE countries. The cow was the offspring of a Dutch dam and a bull of American descent Paul Brown of the NIH announces that intracerebral injection of CJD-infected mice blood can transmit CJD to healthy mice
30 March 1997	A 62-year old man in Indiana dies of CJD. The price of cattle traded on the Chicago Mercantile Exchange down by maximum allowable 1.5 cents to 68.8 cents a pound for April contract. Corn and soybeans also suffered
April 1997	The UK Government admits that it suppressed a list of burial sites of 617 cattle infected with BSE. European and UK guidelines say that carcasses should be incinerated
16 April 1997	USDA restricts importation of meat and by-products from ruminants in the Netherlands
5 June 1997	UK Government announces new control for scrapie which orders all sheep suspected of having the disease to be slaughtered
7 August 1997	US FDA final rule enacted which bans the use of slaughtered animal parts (except pork or horse, and not including blood, gelatin, or milk) in livestock feed. This

rule, effective 4 August 1997, does not apply to pet food, or chicken or hog feed

6 October 1997   Dr Stanley Prusiner awarded the Nobel Prize for Medicine for his discovery of the prion

3 December 1997   On the advice of SEAC the UK Government makes a statement to the effect that they will take action "to require that no beef with the bone in from cattle over 6 months old should be sold to the consumer".

Compiled by Veronica Demko from a variety of sources, including: *BSE, A Chronology of Events*, from the MAFF web page: www.maff.gov.uk/animalh/ bse/chron/htm; *Bovine Spongiform Encephalopathy (BSE)* Fact sheet N113, from the WHO www.who.ch/programmes/emc/bse.facts.htm; "The Beef About BSE and US Food Safety" published by International Food Information Council Foundation, Washington, DC; with contributions by Eve Brouwer.

Appendix 2

Program to Eradicate BSE in the United Kingdom

Kevin Taylor

Executive Summary

1.1. This programme document describes all the measures taken against BSE in the United Kingdom since 1988, together with further measures now being introduced or proposed.

1.2. The objectives of Government action are three-fold:

(a) to protect consumers of bovine products in the UK and elsewhere against any risk, however remote, that BSE may be transmissible to man;
(b) to eradicate BSE in the UK cattle herd; and
(c) to prevent transmission to other animal species.

1.3. Although the primary purpose of this document is to review action aimed at eradicating BSE in cattle, it also presents a full picture of action taken to protect human health.

1.4. There is a detailed explanation of what we know about the nature of BSE. It is unlike other major animal diseases such as foot and mouth disease or swine fever, which are highly contagious. It is one of a group of diseases – transmissible spongiform encephalopathies – which most scientists believe are caused by abnormal forms of protein (prion protein). All evidence so far indicates that in field conditions infection is acquired by consumption of contaminated animal feed, not passed directly from animal to animal. The belief that it can be spread by other means, e.g. maternal transmission remains speculative.

1.5. The two key aims of UK Government action (each supported by a growing body of research evidence) have been:

(a) to exclude from cattle feed all ruminant material which could convey BSE to cattle;
(b) to exclude from the human food chain every bit of those (relatively few) parts of the bovine carcase which, laboratory experiments show, could

convey BSE infectivity, if the animal were infected, and which could convey BSE to man, if it were transmissible to man.

1.6. A large body of rules to achieve these twin aims has been introduced by legislation between June 1988 and May 1996: 57 legal instruments in total.

1.7. Three key features of this legislation are:

(a) progressive steps towards the complete exclusion of mammalian meat and bonemeal (MBM) from all farm animal feed (in its present form this exclusion goes further than the restrictions applicable elsewhere in the EU);
(b) a requirement that all cattle which are suspected of having BSE are slaughtered and destroyed;
(c) a requirement to remove Specified Bovine Offals (SBO; now Specified Bovine Material – SBM) from healthy cattle carcases at the time of slaughter, and to destroy them under strict controls. (These requirements, which are for the protection of human health, are not matched in any other member state where BSE is present.)

1.8. Enforcement of these rules is the responsibility, in Great Britain, of the Ministry of Agriculture, Fisheries and Food (State Veterinary Service and – since April 1995 – the Meat Hygiene Service); and, in Northern Ireland, of the Department of Agriculture (mainly the Veterinary Service). Since 1995, the Meat Hygiene Service has given the national authorities a firmer grip than ever before over enforcement of controls in slaughterhouses, cutting plants and cold stores, and the ability to carry through changes quickly and on a uniform basis throughout Great Britain.

1.9. Systems of enforcement have been progressively tightened in response to the implementation of rules and new scientific evidence. The key responses were:

(a) feed: progressively tighter rules on exclusion of MBM from cattle feed, backed up by new tests for, and procedures for testing, animal feed;
(b) slaughterhouses: progressively stricter rules on removal and destruction of SBM, backed up by uniform and rigorous inspection by Meat Hygiene Service, monitored by the State Veterinary Service.

1.10. Details are given of the large program of research in the UK designed to add to our knowledge of how BSE behaves, as a basis both for well targeted action to eradicate it in cattle and for taking appropriate and proportionate action to protect humans against any risk it may present. Research is also directed towards the development of a test which can identify infected cattle whilst still alive, and to improve post-mortem diagnostic tests.

1.11. Government expenditure on combating BSE, by March 1996, had reached £150m (180m ecu) on compensation to farmers and destruction of 190,000 cattle suspected of BSE (160,000 confirmed cases); £52m (63m ecu) on research; and £35m (43m ecu) on administering controls specifically against

BSE. For 1996–7 the budget for research on BSE has been increased by £1m to £9m, and the Meat Hygiene Service budget has been increased by £39 million specifically for additional controls in slaughterhouses.

1.12. The measures described have had a clear impact. As BSE has an incubation period of about 5 years, it was expected that action taken in 1988–90 would take some years to show through. Evidence of this is presented.

BSE in the UK cattle herd is now demonstrably in sharp decline, having fallen 67 per cent from a peak in 1992–3: numbers of confirmed cases:

	Number	Percentage of herd
1992	36,681	0.3
1993	34,370	0.3
1994	23,944	0.2
1995	14,076	0.1
1996 (estimated)	8,000	0.07

(To set these figures in context, the UK cattle herd numbers approximately 11.5 million.)

1.13. The immediate response to the announcement in March 1996 of a possible link between BSE and CJD, SEAC's advice at that stage, and the crisis in consumer confidence, was:

(i)   a total ban on use of MBM in all farm animal feed – thereby going beyond EU rules, to ensure that *no* cross-contamination of cattle feed is possible;
(ii) the whole head of bovine animals now proscribed as SBM;
(iii) an increase in the Meat Hygiene Service budget noted above (thereby doubling the agency's total budget);
(iv) a ban on sale for human consumption of meat from cattle over 30 months old (cases of BSE are very rare in cattle below this age);
(v)   the slaughter, rendering and incineration of all bovine animals over 30 months at the end of their useful lives. This has resulted in the slaughter of over 60,000 animals since May 1996, and the total will reach 1 million in the first year of operation.

1.14. Further measures now in preparation or proposed are:

(i)   an improved system of identifying cattle and recording their movements, to be introduced by stages, starting in July 1996;
(ii) a scheme for registering and tightly controlling specialist beef herds, with a long record of freedom from BSE; to be launched in June/July 1996;
(iii) selective culling during 1996 of cattle most at risk of BSE (see 1.19).

1.15. Action on animal feed is still believed to be the most effective way of eradicating BSE. Evidence still strongly supports the view that BSE is spread through feed; and that controls applied in the UK to date have had less impact than intended because of incomplete compliance, not because the measures themselves were misconceived. Government intends to fund a scheme to recall from manufacturers and farms residual stocks of feed that might contain meat and bonemeal, so as to ensure 100 per cent compliance with the new stricter rules made in March; and this will be followed within a few weeks by a complete legal ban on holding any such feed.

1.16. A cohort study of maternal transmission will be completed early in 1997. Other studies have found no evidence that BSE is transmitted this way, and there is at present no basis for acting as if it were.

1.17. There are suggestions that all cattle in herds where BSE occurs should be slaughtered. But the scientific evidence strongly indicates that this is not the way to eradicate BSE from the British herd; and evidence from countries where this policy is followed is against it: whole herd slaughter has had no measurable impact on the incidence of BSE in the countries which have followed such a policy.

1.18. The UK is, however, intending to introduce a scheme for *selective* culling of up to 80,000 cattle which can be identified as at particularly high risk of BSE. The cattle would be selected from three year-classes in which BSE is most likely to arise, and further selected on the basis of likely exposure to contaminated feed along with cattle known to have contracted BSE. Details are given on the action proposed, with supporting scientific justification. This would be subject to approval by Parliament. It could reduce the number of BSE cases in 1996 by between 15 and 30 per cent over and above the year-on-year decline of around 40 per cent which is being achieved by the measures already in place.

1.19. The paper concludes that eradication of BSE in the UK will be achieved by the policies already in force, and rigorous enforcement of them on farms, in slaughterhouses, at rendering plants and in feed mills. Rules are now in place to achieve that, and beyond the feed recall scheme, soon to be operated, it is hard to see how the system could be made any more effective.

Decline of the disease could be accelerated by carefully selected culling, firmly based on what is known about BSE and how it is transmitted. This action is recommended.

Culling going beyond this would not be cost-effective or proportionate to the impact achievable and, taking account of other measures in force for the protection of the public in the UK, does not appear to be justified.

1.20. The UK Government firmly believes that it has a coherent, rigorous and scientifically justified strategy for eradicating BSE and protecting human health. We already have in place measures to protect both public and animal health along the lines recommended by OIE at its May 1996 meeting. Banning the feed which causes the disease is demonstrably eradicating BSE. Banning from human food any material which could harbour infectivity is a full safeguard for human health. There is no scientific evidence that British beef in 1996 is anything but safe to eat.

London
31 May 1996

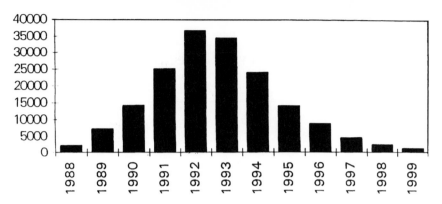

Number of confirmed cases per year, including predicted figures for 1996–9 on the basis of current policy

Meat Hygiene Service: Specified Bovine Material Controls

What is SBM?

Specified Bovine Material includes the head (including the brain, but excluding the tongue), spinal cord, spleen, thymus, tonsils and intestines of bovine animals over six months of age. These tissues are required to be removed from the human and animal food chains because our knowledge of BSE and other transmissible spongiform encephalopathies indicates that they are the tissues most likely to harbour infectivity.

The Legislation

There has been legislation relating to the banning of specified bovine offals since November 1989. The current legislation applying to SBM is *The Specified Bovine Material (No. 2) Order 1996.* The provisions of that Order are central to the protection of public and animal health by removing any potential sources of infectivity from the animal food chain. It requires the removal of all SBM from all cattle at slaughter.

Compliance with these controls is of paramount importance. In the light of recent developments on BSE and the resultant crisis in market confidence in beef, the SBM controls in slaughterhouses effectively underpin the Government's strategies not only to eradicate BSE and to protect public health, but also to retain consumer confidence in beef in the UK and to restore our beef and beef product export markets.

Controls in Slaughterhouses

The MHS provides constant supervision, in the slaughterhall, during the slaughter and dressing of all bovine animals which are eligible for human consumption by virtue of being less than 30 months of age. This supervision includes:

(a) frequent monitoring of the removal, staining and disposal of the spinal cord in accordance with the legislation;

(b) frequent monitoring of the removal by trimming or washing of all debris within the vertebral canal which might contain any spinal cord;

(c) a detailed final inspection of every carcase before it is stamped to ensure that after the completion of dressing all visible traces of spinal cord have been removed from the spinal canal together with any debris that might obscure the spinal cord and there is no visible evidence of contamination by SBM on any part of the carcase.

The consumption of meat from animals over 30 months has been banned.

What is the MHS Doing to Enforce the New SBM Controls?

The MHS is well placed as a national organisation to enforce the SBM controls rigorously, comprehensively, and consistently. It is fully committed to ensuring that industry complies 100% with the new regulations, and to ensure that sufficient MHS staff are available to enforce these important public health controls. The Government has made substantial additional funds available to enable the MHS to do this.

WHO **Fact Sheet N113: (Revised) April 1996**

Bovine Spongiform Encephalopathy (BSE)

Bovine spongiform encephalopathy (BSE) first came to the attention of the scientific community in November 1986 with the appearance in cattle of a newly recognized form of neurological disease in the United Kingdom. Between November 1986 and May 1995 approximately 150,000 cases of this newly recognized cattle disease were confirmed from approximately 33,500 herds of cattle in the UK. Epidemiological studies in the UK at that time suggested that the source of disease was cattle feed prepared from carcasses of dead ruminants, and that changes in the process of preparing cattle feed introduced in 1981–2 may have been a risk factor. Speculation as to the cause of the appearance of the disease in the food chain of cattle has ranged from spontaneous occurrence in cattle, the carcasses of which then entered the cattle food chain; to entry into the cattle food chain from the carcasses of sheep with a similar disease.

BSE is associated with a transmissible agent, the nature of which is not yet fully understood. The agent affects the brain and spinal cord of cattle and lesions are characterized by sponge-like changes visible with an ordinary microscope. It is a highly stable agent, resisting heating at normal cooking temperatures and to even higher temperatures such as those used for pasteurization, sterilization at usual temperatures and times, as well as to freezing and drying. The disease is fatal for cattle within weeks to months of its onset.

By May 1995, BSE had been reported from ten countries and areas outside the UK. In one group of countries – France, Portugal, Republic of Ireland and Switzerland – the disease occurred in native cattle, and this was thought to be in part related to importation of cattle feed from the UK. In another group – Falkland Islands (Las Malvinas), Oman Sultanate, Germany, Canada, Italy and Denmark – cases were only identified in cattle imported from the UK.

In July 1988 the UK banned the use of ruminant proteins in the preparation of cattle feed, and in November 1989 the UK banned the use of brain and spinal cord – as well as tonsil, thymus, spleen and intestine – of cattle origin (known as Specified Bovine Offals or SBOs) in foods for human consumption. Cattle are continuously monitored for BSE in all affected countries, and BSE is decreasing in the UK.

BSE is one of several different forms of transmissible brain disease of animals. Others include scrapie, a disease common in sheep; a similar neurological disease in animals such as the mink, and in North America in mule deer and elk; and, recently, neurological disease in household cats, and in captive bovine and feline species, the majority of which appear to have been in the UK.

Diseases in humans with sponge-like findings in brain under the microscope, and with severe and fatal neurological signs and symptoms, include kuru, a disease which appears to be transmitted by human ritual handling of bodies and brains of the dead; and Creutzfeldt–Jakob disease (CJD). CJD occurs in a form associated with a hereditary predisposition (approximately 10 per cent of cases); and in a more common, sporadic form that accounts for the remaining 90 per cent. In recent years, it has been shown that CJD can be transmitted to humans by treatment with natural human growth hormone or grafting of tissues surrounding human brain, and these means of transmission have now been controlled in the industrialized countries where these procedures were practised. Another similar human disease is Gerstmann–Sträussler–Schenker (GSS) syndrome which appears to be familial, occurring in persons with an apparent hereditary predisposition.

After the identification of BSE, and as a regular activity to continue the study of the possible hazards of BSE for humans, WHO held three meetings on the spongiform encephalopathies in 1991, 1993 and 1995; and one in collaboration with the Office of International Epizootics in 1994. The purpose of these meetings was to review the existing state of knowledge on spongiform encephalopathies including BSE, to evaluate possible means of transmission, and to identify risk factors for infection. An express purpose of these meetings was to review the possible human public health implications of animal spongiform encephalopathies, with special emphasis on BSE.

The most recent WHO meeting compared the annual number of cases of CJD in France, Germany, Italy, Netherlands and the UK. This comparison showed that rates were similar in all these countries (approximately one per million), as was the age distribution and duration of illness prior to death, and conclusions of this meeting were that the epidemiological evidence in Europe did not indicate a change in the incidence of CJD that could be attributed to BSE. Cases reported from the UK were those which were identified through routine reporting and from an intensified surveillance system for CJD-like illness which had been set up in 1990.

A newly recognized variant form of CJD was identified in ten patients in the UK during the 12-month period after this most recent WHO meeting and was first reported by the United Kingdom in March 1996. In contrast to typical cases of sporadic CJD, this variant form affected young patients (mean age 26.3 years) with a relatively long duration of illness (mean 14.1 months).

The characteristic neuropathological profile in this variant consists of numerous widespread kuru-type amyloid plaques with surrounding vacuolation and severe cerebellar lesions. No abnormalities in the prion protein gene have been demonstrated so far in any of the cases.

Case Definition for v-CJD

To date, so far all patients identified in the UK who have died were 41 years of age or less. A suspect case shows the following clinical features:

(a) a psychiatric presentation with anxiety, depression, withdrawal and other behavioural changes with progression to neurological abnormalities;
(b) onset of a progressive cerebellar syndrome within weeks or months of presentation;
(c) forgetfulness and other memory impairment, with dementia in the late stages;
(d) myoclonus in the late stages.

The EEG does not show the changes normally observed in classical CJD. Less common features include early onset of dyasesthesia in limbs and face at presentation, and chorea, extrapyramidal and pyramidal signs later in the illness. Neuropathological diagnosis is mandatory for confirmation of suspect v-CJD cases. Confirmatory examination of the brain should show the following neuropathological features:

(a) numerous widespread kuru-type amyloid plaques surrounded by vacuoles;
(b) spongiform change most evident in the basal ganglia and thalamus;
(c) prion protein accumulation in high density shown by immunocyto-chemistry, particularly in the cerebellum.

At present there have been ten cases of v-CJD reported in the UK and one case reported in France; its geographical distribution, however, needs to be better defined.

A link has not been proven between v-CJD and the effect of exposure to the BSE agent, although this is the most likely hypothesis. Further data are urgently required from scientific studies on these variant cases. More retrospective and prospective monitoring and surveillance studies on all forms of CJD, modelled on current European collaborative studies, are required throughout the world.

At a consultation organized by WHO on 2–3 April 1996, the following recommendations for the protection of public health were made:

(a) No part or product of any animal which has shown signs of a TSE should enter any food chain (human or animal). In particular:
   (i) all countries must ensure the killing and safe disposal of all parts or products of such animals so that TSE infectivity can not enter any food chain;

     (ii) all countries should review their rendering procedures to ensure that they effectively inactivate TSE agents.

(b)   All countries should establish continuous surveillance and compulsory notification for BSE according to the recommendations of the *International Animal Health Code* of the Office International des Epizooties (OIE).

     In the absence of surveillance data the status of a country with respect to the occurrence of BSE must be considered as unknown.

(c)   Countries should not permit tissues that are likely to contain the BSE agent to enter any food chain (human or animal).

(d)   All countries should ban the use of ruminant tissues in ruminant feed.

(e)   With respect to specific products:

     (i) Milk and milk products, even in countries with a high incidence of BSE, are considered safe. There is evidence from other animal and human spongiform encephalopathies to suggest that milk does not transmit these diseases.

     (ii) Gelatin in the food chain is considered to be safe if produced by a manufacturing process utilizing production conditions which has been demonstrated to significantly inactivate any residual infectivity that may have been present in source tissues. Tallow is likewise considered safe if effective rendering procedures are in place.

(f)   The risk, if any, of exposure to the BSE agent in countries other than UK is considered lower than in UK. Exposure to the BSE agent in UK was likely to be higher prior to the current BSE regulations. More studies are required to allow a full risk assessment. Incomplete risk assessment hinders accurate risk communication and perception.

     The risks at present associated with exposure to the BSE agent from beef and beef products will be minimized if the recommendations of the present group are implemented.

(g)   Risks from medicinal products and medical devices containing bovine tissues. The importance of obtaining bovine materials destined for the pharmaceutical industry only from countries which have a surveillance system in place and which report either no or only sporadic cases of BSE is reiterated.

     Removal and inactivation procedures contribute to the reduction of the risk of infection but it must be recognized that the BSE agent is remarkably resistant to physicochemical procedures which destroy the infectivity of common micro-organisms.

     (i) Measures recommended to national health authorities to minimize the risk of transmitting the agent causing bovine spongiform encephalopathy via medicinal products, in particular parenteral products, which were developed at the WHO Consultation in 1991 (*Bulletin of the World Health Organization*, 1992; **70**, 183–90) continue to be generally applicable.

     (ii) It is recommended that these measures be reviewed and, if necessary, strengthened, as more information becomes available.

(h) Research on TSE should be promoted especially as regards rapid diagnosis, agent characterisation, and epidemiology of TSEs in humans and animals.

For further information, please contact Health Communications and Public Relations, WHO, Geneva, Telephone (41 22) 791 2535; Fax (41 22) 791 4858.

All WHO Press Releases, Fact Sheets and Features can be obtained on Internet on the WHO home page http://www.who.ch/

Appendix 5

World Health Organization: Emerging and Other Communicable Diseases (EMC)

Report of a WHO Consultation on Public Health Issues related to Human and Animal Transmissible Spongiform Encephalopathies

With the participation of FAO and OIE

Geneva, Switzerland
2–3 April 1996

1. Introduction

During a Consultation on Transmissible Spongiform Encephalopathies (TSEs), which was convened in Geneva on 2–3 April 1996, a group of international experts reviewed the public health issues related to bovine spongiform encephalopathy (BSE) and the emergence of a new variant of Creutzfeldt–Jakob disease (v-CJD) in humans, as officially reported by the United Kingdom on 20 March 1996, and made recommendations for the protection of public health.

The Consultation was opened by Dr H. Nakajima, Director-General of WHO. He stressed the fact that the possible association between BSE and CJD or its variant once again raised concern about the ability of an infectious agent to cross the species barrier between animals and humans, as in the case of salmonella, plague, hantavirus, and many other zoonotic diseases.

This Consultation was the fourth organized by WHO on the TSEs since 1991. It reviewed the report of the previous WHO Consultation held on 17–19 May 1995 (document WHO/CDS/VPH/95.145) in the light of recently acquired scientific and clinical findings on BSE and other spongiform encephalopathies, including the newly reported human spongiform encephalopathy.

Drs J. Losos (Canada) and J. Gibbs (US) were chairpersons of the Consultation and Dr H. Longbottom (Australia) was rapporteur.

2. Bovine Spongiform Encephalopathy

2.1 Background

1. BSE is a transmissible spongiform encephalopathy (TSE) of cattle which was first identified in the UK in 1986. TSE is a term for a group of diseases

associated with a transmissible agent, the nature of which is not fully known. The agent displays many virus-like features, such as strain variation and mutation, but differs from conventional viruses in being exceptionally resistant to heat, ultraviolet and ionizing radiation, and to chemical disinfectants.

Transmission of BSE to cattle appears to have been via contaminated meat and bonemeal in concentrate feed (sheep or cattle may have been the original source of the agent).

The epidemic in the UK (the only country with a high incidence of the disease) appears to have been due mainly to the recycling of affected bovine material back to cattle before the July 1988 ruminant feed ban became effective.

To date there is no firm evidence to suggest that either maternal or horizontal transmission occurs. It is noted that no closed herd study has been undertaken to clarify these aspects but a cohort study is under way and will be completed early in 1997.

The incidence of the disease is declining significantly in the UK, although the measures introduced have not so far brought the epidemic to a halt.

2. The full geographical distribution of BSE is incompletely known. BSE in native cattle has also been identified and reported at a much lower incidence than in the UK in four other European countries.

In these latter countries epidemiological investigations indicate that only some of the BSE cases in native cattle could be proven to be related to consumption of feed which might have been contaminated with the BSE agent.

2.2 Recommendations for the Protection of Public Health

1. No part or product of any animal which has shown signs of a TSE should enter any food chain (human or animal). In particular all countries must ensure the killing and safe disposal of all parts or products of such animals so that TSE infectivity can not enter any food chain. All countries should review their rendering procedures to ensure that they effectively inactivate TSE agents.

2. All countries should establish continuous surveillance and compulsory notification for BSE according to the recommendations of the *International Animal Health Code* of the Office International des Epizooties (OIE).

In the absence of surveillance data the status of a country with respect to the occurrence of BSE must be considered unknown.

3. Countries should not permit tissues that are likely to contain the BSE agent to enter any food chain (human or animal).

4. All countries should ban the use of ruminant tissues in ruminant feed.

5. With respect to specific products: milk and milk products, even in countries with a high incidence of BSE, are considered safe. There is evidence from other animal and human spongiform encephalopathies to suggest that milk does not transmit these diseases. Gelatin in the food chain is considered to be safe if

produced by a manufacturing process utilizing production conditions which have been demonstrated to significantly inactivate any residual infectivity (selected references: Annex 1) that may have been present in source tissues. Tallow is likewise considered safe if effective rendering procedures are in place (selected references: Annex 1).

6. The risk, if any, of exposure to the BSE agent in countries other than UK is considered lower than in UK. Exposure to the BSE agent in UK was likely to be higher prior to the current BSE regulations. More studies are required to allow a full risk assessment. Incomplete risk assessment hinders accurate risk communication and perception.

The risks at present associated with exposure to the BSE agent from beef and beef products will be minimized if the recommendations of the present group are implemented.

7. Risks from medicinal products and medical devices containing bovine tissues: the importance is reiterated of obtaining bovine materials destined for the pharmaceutical industry only from countries which have a surveillance system in place and which report either no or only sporadic cases of BSE. Removal and inactivation procedures contribute to the reduction of the risk of infection but it must be recognized that the BSE agent is remarkably resistant to physicochemical procedures which destroy the infectivity of common micro-organisms. Measures recommended to national health authorities to minimize the risk of transmitting the agent causing bovine spongiform encephalopathy via medicinal products, in particular parenteral products, which were developed at the WHO Consultation in 1991 (*Bulletin of the World Heath Organization*, 1992, **70**: 183–190) continue to be generally applicable. It is recommended that these measures be reviewed and, if necessary, strengthened as more information becomes available.

8. Research on TSE should be promoted, especially regarding rapid diagnosis, agent characterization, and epidemiology of TSEs in humans and animals.

3. A New Variant of Creutzfeldt–Jakob Disease (v-CJD)

3.1 Background

1. TSEs in humans include CJD (which may occur in sporadic, inherited, and iatrogenic forms), Gerstmann–Sträussler–Scheinker syndrome and fatal familial insomnia (both of which are inherited disorders), and kuru, a disorder which was associated with ritualistic cannibalism in Papua New Guinea.

A newly recognized variant form of CJD (v-CJD) has been identified in ten patients in the UK. In contrast to typical cases of sporadic CJD, this variant form has affected young patients (mean age 26.3 years) with a relatively long duration of illness (mean 14.1 months).

The characteristic neuropathological profile in this variant consists of numerous widespread kuru-type amyloid plaques with surrounding vacuolation and severe cerebellar lesions. No abnormalities in the prion protein gene have been demonstrated so far in any of the cases.

2. Case definition for v-CJD. To date, all patients identified in the UK who died of the disease were 41 years of age or less. A suspect case shows the following clinical features:

(a) a psychiatric presentation with anxiety, depression, withdrawal and other behavioural changes with progression to neurological abnormalities;
(b) onset of a progressive cerebellar syndrome within weeks or months of presentation;
(c) forgetfulness and other memory impairment, with dementia in the late stages;
(d) myoclonus in the late stages;
(e) the EEG does not show the changes normally observed in classical CJD.

Less common features include early onset of dysaesthesia in limbs and face at presentation, and chorea, extrapyramidal and pyramidal signs later in the illness.

Neuropathological diagnosis is *mandatory* for confirmation of suspected v-CJD cases.

Confirmatory examination of the brain should show the following neuropathological features:

(a) numerous widespread kuru-type amyloid plaques surrounded by vacuoles;
(b) spongiform change most evident in the basal ganglia and thalamus;
(c) prion protein accumulation in high density shown by immunocyto-chemistry, particularly in the cerebellum.

3.2 Recommendations

1. v-CJD is reported at present only in the UK; its geographical distribution needs to be better defined.

2. A link has not yet been proven between v-CJD in the UK and the effect of exposure to the BSE agent.

The most likely hypothesis for v-CJD is the exposure of the UK population to BSE; further data are urgently required from scientific studies on these variant cases. More retrospective and prospective monitoring and surveillance studies on all forms of CJD, modelled on current European collaborative studies, are required throughout the world.

Annex 1

Brown, P., R.G. Rohwer & D.C. Gajdusek 1986. Newer data on the inactivation of scrapie virus or Creutzfeldt–Jakob disease virus in brain tissue. *Journal of Infectious Diseases* **153**, 1145–8.

Di Martino, A., J. Safar, M. Ceroni & C.J. Gibbs jun. 1992. Purification of non-infectious ganglioside preparations from scrapie-infected brain tissue. *Archives of Virology* **124**, 111–21.

Diringer, H. & R.H. Kimberlin 1983. Infectious scrapie agent is not as small as recent claims suggest. *Bioscience Reports* **3**, 563–8.

Hunter, G.D. & G.C. Millson 1964. Studies on the heat stability and chromatographic behaviour of the scrapie agent. *Journal of General Microbiology* **37**, 251–8.

Hunter, G.D. 1965. Progress toward the isolation and characterisation of the scrapie agent. In *Slow, Latent and Temperate Virus Infections* D.C. Gajdusek, C.J. Gibbs, jun. & M. Alpers (eds). NINDB Monograph No. 2, 259–62. US Government Printing Office, Washington, DC.

Kimberlin, R.H., G.C. Millson & G.D. Hunter 1971. An experimental examination of the scrapie agent in cell membrane mixtures. III. Studies of the operational size of the scrapie agent. *Journal of Comparative Pathology* **81**, 383–91.

Marsh, R.F. & R.P. Hanson 1969. Physical and chemical properties of the transmissible mink encephalopathy agent. *Journal of Virology* **3**, 176–80.

Millson, G.C., G.D. Hunter & R.H. Kimberlin 1976. The physio-chemical nature of the scrapie agent. In *Slow Virus Diseases of Animals and Man* R.H. Kimberlin (ed.), ch. 11, pp. 243–66, North-Holland, Amsterdam.

Pocchiari, M., G. Macchi, S. Peano & A. Conz 1988. Can potential hazard of Creutzfeldt–Jakob disease infectivity be reduced in the production of human growth hormone? Inactivation experiments with the 263K strain of scrapie. *Archives of Virology* **98**, 131–5.

Pocchiari, M., S. Peano, A. Gonz, A. Eshkol, F. Maillard, P. Brown, C.J. Gibbs, jun., Y.G. Xi, E. Tenham-Fisher & G. Macchi 1991. Combination ultrafiltration and 6M urea treatment of human growth hormone effectively minimizes risk from potential Creutzfeldt–Jakob disease virus contamination *Hormone Research* **35**, 161–6.

Taguchi, F., Y. Tamai, K. Uchida, R. Kitajima, H. Kojima, T. Kawaguchi, Y. Ohtani & S. Miura 1991. Proposal for a procedure for complete inactivation of the Creutzfeldt–Jakob disease agent. *Archives of Virology* **119**, 297–301.

Tamai, Y., F. Taguchi & S. Miura 1988. Inactivation of the Creutzfeldt–Jakob disease agent. *Annals of Neurology* **24**, 466–7.

Taylor, D.M., A.G. Dickinson, H. Fraser, P.A. Robertson, P.R. Salacinski & P.J. Lowry 1985. Preparation of growth hormone free from contamination with unconventional slow viruses. *Lancet* **ii**, 260–2.

Taylor, D.M., H. Fraser, L. McConnell, D.A. Brown, K.L. Brown, K.A. Lamza, G.R.A. Smith 1994. Decontamination studies with the agents of bovine spongiform encephalopathy and scrapie. *Archives of Virology* **139**, 313–26.

Afterword

In 1906, Upton Sinclair's novel, *The Jungle*, prompted discussions on the safety of the food supply and the nature of working conditions in the United States. The documentary novel prompted President Theodore Roosevelt to spit out his breakfast sausage in January 1906 and invite Sinclair to the White House. The ire of the whole nation contributed enormously to the landmark passage of the Pure Food and Drug Act of 1906. Sixty-one years later, Sinclair watched President Lyndon Johnson sign the Wholesome Meat Act of 1967.

Ninety years after Sinclair's novel, the British Government's SEAC report prompted another kind of political and public outcry. Many political decisions surrounding BSE are described in *The Mad Cow Crisis: Health and the Public Good*, from the banning of British beef, to the non-cooperation policy reminiscent of the French boycott some thirty years ago. The public reaction included McDonalds' decision to suspend the use of British beef, and even USA talk show host Oprah Winfrey's public disclosure that she would not eat beef because of mad cow disease, which sent the Commodity Exchange down the maximum allowable amount in one day. As this book goes to press, there are many questions still being resolved: will there be a European version of the Food and Drug Administration? Will there be regulation on all products (including gelatin in pharmaceutical preparations) available in the European region? And, is there any preparation or mechanism in place to avert future crises?

In the United States, there have been some measures to protect the food supply, instituted subsequent to the early phase of the European crisis. In 1996, President Clinton signed an act to create the most stringent regulations on the beef industry in US history. In June 1997, the Food and Drug Administration issued a regulation instituting a mammal-to-ruminant feed ban. Research is also being conducted on the culling techniques that might also be somehow linked to human disease.

During the preparation of this book, I have reviewed countless documents and publications, attended conferences, and monitored developments in the epidemiology and science of BSE and CJD. A recent issue of the *British Medical Journal* (15 August 1997) presented data from Dr Bob Will of the CJD surveillance unit in Edinburgh and colleagues from the London School of Hygiene and Tropical Medicine. They concluded the increased reports of CJD since the early 1980s appear to reflect better methods of monitoring the disease, rather than true changes in incidence. The worldwide incidence of any type of CJD is still constant at one in one million, even adding the identification of v-CJD. It is important to note that as this book goes to print, there has been no increase in the incidence of CJD cases since the March 1996 announcement.

While this book was under development, we have witnessed the testing of scientific discoveries. In October 1997, the Nobel Prize for Medicine was awarded to Dr Stanley Prusiner for discovering and naming prions. Hypotheses for diagnosing prion diseases in cattle were proclaimed and subsequently refuted in scientific studies.

As of this date, I stand by my initial editorial in the *Boston Globe* (6 April 1996), the *Financial Times* (21 October 1996) and the *Wall Street Journal* (12 May 1997). I continue to examine the sensationalist books that proclaim a crisis of epidemic proportion. Today, the facts are the same, with three important questions still left unanswered:

1. Why has the infectivity never been detected in muscle or milk from animals naturally infected with BSE or any other spongiform encephalopathy?
2. If BSE can be transmitted to humans in the form of CJD, what is the natural vector between species (as meat and milk are the most widely consumed bovine products)?
3. Why have these new variant cases that are purportedly "linked" occurred principally in young people, even though bovine products are equally consumed among all age segments of the British population?

As I review the coverage of other health scares, I find that there are similar examples of miscommunication by "officials" that erode our faith in the system rather than help evoke inquiry and understanding for a healthier public. For example, in the summer of 1997, the largest recall in US history of ground beef products – over 25 million pounds of hamburger meat – occurred due to an *E. Coli* bacteria threat. While it might be appropriate to take precautions on ingesting tainted food, inappropriate statements are worrisome. For example, a proclamation by Michael Osterhom, Minnesota State epidemiologist that "[Eating rare hamburgers] is like driving without a seat belt at 90 miles per hour and going through red lights"[1] alarmed the public. This book explores how such overblown proclamations of risk cause more harm than good.

The Mad Cow Crisis: health and the public good challenges us to take an important role as members of society. The onus is on those who have the ability to balance sense with science, so that we avoid science without sense. Perhaps we should heed the words of Galileo Galilei, who himself had issues with the beliefs of his time: "In questions of science, the authority of a thousand is not worth the humble reasoning of a single individual."[2]

Scott C. Ratzan
October 1997

Notes

1 Martha Groves. Beef recall expansion sparks fears. 16 August 1997. p. A22. *Los Angeles Times.*
2 Galileo Galilei In *The Forbes Book of Business Quotations* Ted Goodman (ed.) (1997) Black Dog and Levinthal Publishers, New York, 737.

Notes on Contributors

Paul Anand, D.Phil. (Oxon), M.Sc., is Reader in Decision Theory at De Montfort University, Milton Keynes. He has previously held posts at the universities of Oxford, Cambridge and York. He specializes in research on the foundations and applications of decision theory and is the author of *Foundations of Rational Choice Under Risk*. He is currently managing editor of *Risk, Decision and Policy* and works on a variety of topics including AIDS, government administration and the Internet.

Eve Brouwer is manager of the Campus Division of the National Safety Council and serves as the Council's link to environmental health and safety offices at colleges and universities worldwide. She is also the Council's representative to the National Council on Aging and to the Risk Watch Coalition. She has contributed, as general consultant, writer and editor, to *A Child's First Library of Learning Health and Safety, Safety in the Science Classroom* and to the SafeLife Curriculum, an educational program run by the National Safety Council.

Michael Chamberlain, Ph.D., is a journalist, publisher and communications specialist with a professional career in newspapers, business and consumer magazines, radio and television on both sides of the Atlantic spanning nearly 30 years. In 1993 he was awarded his Ph.D. in Communication at Florida State University, where he specialized in multimedia publishing and new media technologies. He lectured at Florida State University and was a visiting professor in Communication Studies at Emerson College, Boston, before returning to the UK to become Director, New Media Activities, for United News and Media plc, with a worldwide brief covering 600 publications in three continents. In 1996 he joined the board of specialist new media consultancy Informed Sources International. He has contributed to various books and academic journals and a joint paper *Problems of Diffusion in High Technology* won the open section at the Broadcast Education Association convention in 1993.

Lester M. Crawford, DVM, Ph.D., is Director of the Georgetown Center for Food and Nutrition Policy. Previously, he was Executive Director of the

Association of American Veterinary Medical Colleges in Washington DC, Executive Vice-President of the National Food Processors Association and Administrator of the US Food Safety and Inspection Service. Earlier he was Director of FDA's Center for Veterinary Medicine. He also served as Head of the Department of Physiology and Pharmacology at the University of Georgia and as a Fellow at the Georgetown University Center for Food and Nutrition Policy. He has just completed a four-year term on the US Food Advisory Committee.

Stephen F. Dealler, MB, Ch.B. MRCPath, is a consultant microbiologist at Burnley General Hospital in the UK. He is particularly known for his work into the safety of modern food which has included research on the food-borne nature of the major UK outbreak of listeriosis, and on the reason why microwave ovens are often unable to kill the bacteria present in food. He was responsible for releasing the epidemiological date indicating that the risk being taken with BSE in the UK was unacceptably high. In 1996 he published a book, *Lethal Legacy*, in which he argued that it is difficult for governments to take action on such a problem as BSE and that responsibility for handling the crisis must be taken by individuals. His current activities include compiling the information for the Internet site on BSE, running the Spongiform Encephalopathy Research Campaign and carrying out research into potential methods of treatment and diagnosis for the disease.

Veronica Demko is a Masters candidate in the Emerson-Tufts program in Health Communication. She previously worked as a community development volunteer in the US Peace Corps in Niger, West Africa. Since 1996, she has been Research Fellow in Health Communication at Emerson College, examining the role of the media in the development of the mad cow crisis. She also serves as assistant to the editor for the textbook entitled *Principles of Health Communication*, due to be published in 1999.

Daniel Dornbusch is a Masters candidate in the Emerson-Tufts program in Health Communication, a consultant in the biotechnology industry and assistant producer and co-host of a cable television program addressing health issues. He is also president and CEO of Digital Genetics, Inc, a company that develops software for genetic research.

Marcie Everett-Weber is Director of Corporate Communications at Centrepoint Technologies in Ottawa, and co-founder of the Hopkins & Weber Communications team, with Dawn Hopkins. The team's projects have included developing a pan-European communications agenda for the World Wide Fund for Nature, suggesting solutions to issues managing cultural diversity at NATO and analyzing gender communication issues at international women's conferences.

Catherine C.A. Goethals, Cand., lic, Philology in Germanic Languages postgrad, is Coordinator of the Communications Office at the College of Europe. With a Masters degree in Multilingual Business Communication, she has been actively involved in several TEMPUS and PHARE programs, introducing students of central and east European countries to EU terminology. She has also organized and taught workshops on intercultural negotiation and the language and body-language of politicians.

Terri L. Harpold, MD, is currently serving a clinical fellowship in Pediatric Neurosurgery at Children's Hospital of Los Angeles, an affiliate of the University of Southern California. Her areas of interest include the application of advanced imaging techniques and three-dimensional visualization to neurosurgery.

Dawn Hopkins is Communications Consultant for Hopkins & Weber Communications, which she co-founded with Marcie Everett-Weber. She is a published poet, who lives in Nashville.

Simon Hughes was elected as the youngest opposition MP in 1983. He was re-elected for the Southwark and Bermondsey constituency in 1983, 1987 and 1992. After studying law at Selwyn College, Cambridge, he received a postgraduate Certificate in European Studies at the College of Europe in Bruges. He has been the Liberal Democrat spokesperson in parliament on Housing, Health, Environment, Natural Resources and Food, among others. He has jointly authored booklets on human rights, the law and politics, and has introduced many bills in parliament, including those relating to access of information, banning tobacco advertising, and requiring the Queen to pay income taxes. Since November 1995, Mr Hughes has been the party's spokesperson on health and urban policy and he serves as the Liberal Democrat Deputy Whip.

Tim Lang, Ph.D., has been Professor of Food Policy and Director of the Centre for Food Policy at Thames Valley University since March 1994. He was Director of the London Food Commission, 1984–90 and Director of Parents for Safe Food, 1990–94. He has been a food policy advisor to the European Commissioner for the Environment, and advises many local authorities and voluntary bodies. He has been a member of two UK Government Nutrition Taskforce project teams and in 1996 was a consultant to the WHO on BSE and on food policy in the former Soviet Union.

Joan Leach, Ph.D., is Lecturer in Science Communication at Imperial College of Science, Technology and Medicine in London, and the editor of the quarterly journal *Social Epistemology*. She has published on discourse ethics, the history of the role of communicators in science and medicine, and the representation of science in the media during the BSE crisis.

Michael L. Levy, MD, is Assistant Professor of Pediatric Neurological Surgery at the Children's Hospital of Los Angeles, University of Southern California School of Medicine. He also works in the Department of Physiology and Biophysics at the University of Southern California evaluating the relationship of toxins and ribosylation of G-protein on immune response.

Dick Mayon-White, Ph.D., FRCP, FFPHM, is a consultant in communicable disease control for Oxfordshire Health Authority, a senior lecturer at the University of Oxford and a regional epidemiologist in the Public Health Laboratory Service. A local newspaper called him the "crisis doc". His experience ranges from the last-ever outbreak of smallpox, in Birmingham in 1968, through the HIV crisis, the salmonella-in-eggs controversy, vaccine scares and meningitis panics, to the current problems of BSE and chemical pollution incidents.

J. Gregory Payne, Ph.D., is the Chair of the Communication Studies Division of Emerson College. He is an author, speech-writer and expert on political communication, ethics and docudrama. His recent research publications include articles on ethics and the mass media, health communication, and political communication. He has acted as a guest editor for three consecutive special issues of the *American Behavioral Scientist* on US presidential elections, and on political communication.

Scott C. Ratzan, MD, MPA, MA, is Editor in Chief of the *Journal of Health Communication*, Director of the Emerson-Tufts Masters Degree Program in Health Communication, and a Director of the Center for Ethics in Political and Health Communication. He is also Assistant Professor at Emerson College's Division of Communication Studies and Tufts University School of Medicine's Department of Family Medicine and Community Health. Dr Ratzan specializes in health communication, media strategies and negotiation. He has published widely in academic journals and in the international press and has appeared regularly on television to discuss health related issues. He is the editor of *AIDS: Effective Health Communication for the '90s*.

Bradley D. Savage has been a professional in the entertainment industry since 1967 and is currently working in motion picture marketing in Los Angeles.

Ian Wylie, MA (Oxon) Dphil, MIPR, is Head of Communications at the King's Fund where he runs the marketing, press and public relations, publishing and internal communications divisions. He is an advisor to the UK's Department of International Development and regularly works on communications training and consultancy for health authorities and NHS trusts. He has 15 years of experience of public relations in the NHS and in local government. He is author of the NHS Confederation *Guide to Good Communication in NHS Trusts* (1997), as well as a book and essays on the poet and philosopher S. T. Coleridge.

Index

3825